The Support of Breastfeeding

4

Module 1
The Support of Breastfeeding

Rebecca F. Black, MS, RD/LD, IBCLC

Dietitian, Lactation Consultant, Researcher
President, Augusta Nutrition Consultants
Augusta, Georgia

Leasa Jarman, MS

Education Consultant
Augusta, Georgia

Jan Simpson, RN, BSN, IBCLC

Nurse, Lactation Consultant
Tuscaloosa, Alabama

Jones and Bartlett Publishers
Sudbury, Massachusetts

Boston   London   Singapore

Editorial, Sales, and Customer Service Offices

Jones and Bartlett Publishers
40 Tall Pine Drive
Sudbury, MA 01776
508 443-5000
800 832-0034
info@jbpub.com
http://www.jbpub.com

Jones and Bartlett Publishers International
Barb House, Barb Mews
London W6 7PA
UK

Cover illustration is a woodcut print by Russell Wray, Gull Rock Pottery,
325 East Side Road, Hancock, ME 04640.

Acknowledgment: Supported in part through funds from the Georgia WIC Program,
Maternal and Child Health Branch, Division of Public Health, Georgia Department
of Human Resources.

Library of Congress Cataloging-in-Publication Data
The support of breastfeeding / edited by Rebecca F. Black, Leasa Jarman,
   Jan Simpson.
         p.   cm.—(Lactation specialist self-study series : module 1)
      Includes bibliographical references.
      ISBN 0-7637-0208-0 (alk. paper)
      1. Breast feeding—Study and teaching.   I. Black, Rebecca F.
   II. Jarman, Leasa.   III. Simpson, Jan.   IV. Series.
   RJ216.S885   1997
   613.2'69--dc21   97-25569
                                                                          CIP

Editor: Robin Carter
Production Editor: Marilyn E. Rash
Design/Typesetting: Ruth Maassen
Cover Design: Hannus Design Associates
Cover Illustration: Russell Wray
Cover Printing: Malloy Lithographing
Printing and Binding: Malloy Lithographing

Printed in the United States of America
01   00   99   98   97   10   9   8   7   6   5   4   3   2   1

Contents

Preface

Lactation consultants number in the thousands, representing the varied disciplines of counseling, education, nursing, nutrition, occupational therapy, pharmacology, physical therapy, psychology, and medicine. The differing backgrounds of lactation consultants and the lack of a widespread educational program of study for lactation consulting results in professionals with strengths in various areas of lactation. As we enter the next millenium of more control of health-care resources by managed care and less choice by the consumer, it is imperative that those in the lactation consulting profession share a base of knowledge from many disciplines to compete and survive. As resources shrink, health-care professionals must expand their clinical skills to improve their marketability. As boundaries separating prenatal, hospital, and postpartum services are becoming less defined, organizations and hospitals strive to compete for services outside their traditional roles.

This *Lactation Specialist Self-Study Series* draws extensively from the literature of all the disciplines mentioned above. It is designed to be used in four separate modules to present a systematic overview of the profession (Support, Process, Science, and Management of Breastfeeding), emphasizing and reviewing areas for study usually lacking in the academic preparation of nurses and nutritionists. This book, *The Support of Breastfeeding, Module 1*, explores cultural support for and attitudes toward breastfeeding, advantages and hazards of artificial feeding, and breastfeeding support policies and resources.

The three sections in Chapter 1 are devoted to exploring where we are globally in supporting breastfeeding, how cultures evolve or disintegrate in their support of breastfeeding, what impact breastfeeding has on the family and community, and what we can do to prolong lactation both individually and as a community. Emphasis is placed on family-focused, community-based programming to improve breastfeeding incidence, exclusivity, and duration. Information on marketing is provided to help the reader take a systematic approach to supporting breastfeeding at a particular institution or community.

The two sections of Chapter 2 provide an update of what we know about the superiority of human-milk feedings and the inferiority of artificial baby milks, lending support for better informing parents of the differences and heightening the urgency of human milk's importance to our infants. Benefits to the child, parents, and to society and the global community are presented. The increased morbidity and mortality of artificially fed infants is reviewed as are the miscellaneous other risks artificial feeding presents.

Chapter 3's three sections are devoted to exploring the suggested breastfeeding support policies of international and governmental organizations; reviewing the positions on breastfeeding of major health-care organizations; and providing a comprehensive listing of organizations, private companies, government agencies, and so on, that are involved in breastfeeding support. The resource list contains complete mailing information, phone and fax numbers, and e-mail and web site addresses if they are available.

The format of the module is designed to be reader-friendly with pre- and post-test questions for each section and extensive reference lists. *The Support of Breastfeeding* contains 280 multiple-choice questions that are designed to help the learner gauge her or his knowledge prior to and on completion of a section. The format easily lends itself to use in a formal-learning environment, such as an undergraduate or graduate curricula, or for the student or clinician looking for a systematic way to prepare for the profession or obtain continuing education credits.

Acknowledgments

In 1992, the state of Georgia public health nutrition section identified the need to update the knowledge and skills of practicing nurses and nutritionists in the field of lactation. The *Lactation Specialist Self-Study Series* was first developed as an eleven-volume set of modules and was supported in part through funds from the Georgia WIC Program, Maternal and Child Health Branch, Division of Public Health, Georgia Department of Human Resources. Many individuals were instrumental in the early development of the series. I wish to thank Carol McGowan for her vision of the project and the faith that the project would finally come to fruition, Gwen Gustavson for her pilot teaching of the curricula to nutritionists in two health districts in Georgia, and Irene Frei and Frances Wilkinson for their support of the project by providing the needed resources.

Many other individuals have helped this *Series* become a reality: Tracy Howie and Jerry Smith were invaluable for their technical computer expertise; Debi Bocar, Martha Brower, and Julie Stock reviewed all four modules and provided excellent suggestions about them for continuing education applications as well as feedback for improvement; Jatinder Bhatia and Elizabeth Williams also provided valuable constructive feedback from the medical community about selected modules.

I would be remiss if I failed to thank the behind-the-scene supportive individuals who kept my business running for what, at times, must have seemed like forever. Emily Kitchens, my business manager, is invaluable to me and without her organizational abilities, tireless energy, and loyalty Augusta Nutrition Consultants, Inc., would fold. The lactation consultants and peer counselors on staff filled in for me in many situations and provided valuable insight for the *Series*. Many dietetic interns enrolled in the Augusta Area Dietetic Internship combed the library in search of articles as did Donna Wilson. The librarians at the Medical College of Georgia never wearied of my requests for reprints and seemingly daily presence on the Medline. Thanks also goes to the nutrition and pediatric professors at the Medical College of Georgia School of Medicine and Graduate School for their willingness to answer questions and interpret literature.

Jan Simpson, one of the editors, was very instrumental in the *Lactation Specialist Self-Study Series*. Not only did she write several of the chapters but she also helped in the development of the content of the modules as well as the completion of the applications for nursing continuing education credits. Jan and her family worked many hours to get the *Series* finished. Leasa Jarman, another editor, provided expertise on test construction and evaluated each module for completeness of the objectives and each test for accurate measurement of the objectives. Thanks also to the individual contributors who are too numerous to mention here but are all named on the Contributors' list.

I wish to thank my family—Tony, Helen, and Marie—who gave so willingly of Mom and accompanied me on several trips to educational workshops. Many evening hours and weekends were lost to the *Series* and their support was essential to its successful completion. Finally, I wish to acknowledge the presence and guidance of the Lord Jesus Christ who gives me the strength to press on to the prize of eternal life through Him.

Lactation Specialist Self-Study Series

Contributors

Rebecca F. Black, MS, RD/LD, IBCLC
President, Augusta Nutrition
Consultants, Inc.
Augusta, Georgia

Jatinder Bhatia, MBBS
Chief, Section of Neonatology
Medical College of Georgia
Augusta, Georgia

Donna Calhoun, BS, IBCLC
Lactation Consultant
Breast Expressions
Augusta, Georgia

Laurie Cimino, MPH, RD
Public Health Nutritionist
Boone, North Carolina

Jill Goode, MS, RD
Clinical Dietician
Cedar Bluff, Virginia

Bryn Hamilton, RD/LD, IBCLC
Neonatal/Pediatric Dietitian
in Private Practice
Augusta, Georgia

Charlotte Koehler, RNC, CCE, MN, IBCLC
Childbirth Educator and Lactation
Consultant in Private Practice
Fayetteville, North Carolina

Leasa Jarman, MS
Educator
Columbia County School System
Augusta, Georgia

Teresa McCullen, BS, ACCE, IBCLC
Lactation Consultant in Private
Practice
Augusta, Georgia

Robin McRoberts, MS, RD/LD
Public Health Nutritionist
Augusta, Georgia

Jan Simpson, RN, BSN, IBCLC
Lactation Consultant in Private
Practice
Tuscaloosa, Alabama

Richard Simpson, DMD
Pediatric Dentist
Tuscaloosa, Alabama

Betsy Summerfield, BS, MA
Director of Human Resources
Southwestern Community College
Richlands, Virginia

Reviewers

Debi Leslie Bocar, RN, MEd, MS, IBCLC
Oklahoma City, Oklahoma

Martha K. Grodrian, RD, LD, IBCLC
Dayton, Ohio

Pamela D. Hill, PhD, RN
Chicago, Illinois

Kathleen E. Huggins, RN, MS
San Luis Obispo, California

Karen Sanders Moore, RNC, MSN, IBCLC
Saint Louis, Missouri

Julie Stock, MA, IBCLC
Chicago, Illinois

Elizabeth Williams, MD, MPH, IBCLC
Stanford, California

CHAPTER 1

Cultural Support for and Attitudes Toward Breastfeeding

SECTION A

Breastfeeding in Today's Culture

Jill L. Goode, RD/LD
Rebecca F. Black, MS, RD/LD, IBCLC
Betsy E. Summerfield, BS, MBA
Teresa McCullen, BS, IBCLC

LEARNING OBJECTIVES

At the completion of this section, the learner will be able to do the following:

1. Describe the factors that contributed to the rise of the artificial baby milk industry.
2. Discuss the impact of socially determined attitudes on women's choice to breastfeed.
3. Describe the demographics of who breastfeeds in the United States.
4. Differentiate among patterns and trends in infant feeding in the U.S. population as a whole, the WIC population, and the world population.
5. Discuss the factors important in the decision to breastfeed.
6. Describe the barriers to breastfeeding in different population groups.
7. Describe counseling strategies that may be effective in removing barriers.
8. Identify common myths about breastfeeding prevalent in the United States.
9. Write a marketing plan to promote a product or service related to breastfeeding.

OUTLINE

I. History of Artificial Baby Milks

    A. Breastfeeding/artificial baby milks through the ages

    B. Agriculture and medicine endorse artificial baby milks

    C. Industry and lobbyists sustain acceptance of artificial baby milks

    D. Explosion of research into individual and societal benefits from breast-feeding

    E. Feeding of artificial baby milks becomes the norm in the United States

    F. Recognition by medical societies and government that norms must change

II. The Influence of Cultural Mores on Breastfeeding

    A. Reexamining women's liberties as determinants of breastfeeding

    B. Breastfeeding around the globe

        1. Africa

        2. Asia

        3. Europe

        4. Scandinavia

        5. Oceania

        6. Latin America

        7. North America

III. Important Factors in the Decision to Breastfeed

    A. Prenatal education

    B. Perception of benefits

    C. Sociodemographic factors

        1. Parity

        2. Education/marital status/income

        3. Employment

        4. Ethnicity

        5. Maternal age

IV. Factors that Negatively Influence the Decision to Breastfeed

    A. Perception of barriers

    B. Community myths

V. Marketing Breastfeeding

    A. Developing a marketing plan

        1. Purpose and benefits

        2. Past, present, and future use

        3. Internal and external factors to consider in the situational analysis

        4. Identifying the appreciate markets

      5. Segmenting the market

      6. Analyzing alternative opportunities

   B. Steps to implement the marketing plan

      1. Setting goals

      2. Planning and developing strategies

      3. Executing the plan

      4. Effective marketing organization

      5. Analyzing market results

   C. Using the media

      1. Choosing the right mix

      2. Selecting the media mix

      3. Scheduling the advertising

      4. Evaluating the advertising program

PRE-TEST

For questions 1 to 5, choose the best answer.

1. The introduction of foods other than mother's milk to the infant in the first few months of life

   A. began with the practice of wet nursing during the sixteenth century.
   B. is a new practice begun in the twentieth century.
   C. is a result of the artificial baby milk market.
   D. has occurred since pre-Christian times.

2. In the early twentieth century it was not uncommon for doctors

   A. to prescribe individual formulas for babies.
   B. to recommend the feeding of prepackaged artificial baby milks.
   C. to employ wet nurses for hire.
   D. to question the practice of breastfeeding as outdated.

3. Breastfeeding rates were lowest in the United States in the

   A. early fifties.
   B. early eighties.
   C. late forties.
   D. early seventies.

4. Which group leads behavior and social change?

   A. urban poor
   B. urban elite
   C. rural poor
   D. middle class

5. Which of the following is not believed to have contributed to the rise of artificial feeding as the norm in the United States?

   A. greater geographic mobility
   B. increase in small nuclear families

C. decrease in mulitgenerational families

D. increase in breastfeeding role models

For questions 6 to 10, choose the best answer from the following key:

A. 1990   D. 1984

B. 1981   E. 1956

C. 1994

6. The year the United States voted against the WHO Code of Marketing of Breast-milk Substitutes.

7. The year La Leche League International was formed.

8. The year of the first U.S. Surgeon General's Workshop on Breastfeeding and Human Lactation.

9. The year the Innocenti Declaration was adopted at a WHO/UNICEF meeting in Italy.

10. The year the United States voted for the WHO Code of Marketing of Breast-milk Substitutes.

For questions 11 to 15, choose the best answer.

11. Wet nursing was practiced in many cultures for all of the following reasons except to:

   A. create family bonds to prevent marriages.

   B. destroy tribal unity.

   C. promote alliances and make peace with enemy tribes.

   D. free women from a practice that alters body shape.

12. The _____ the maternal income, the _____ the incidence of breastfeeding in the United States.

   A. higher, lower

   B. lower, higher

   C. lower, lower

   D. higher, higher

13. The _____ education, the _____ the incidence of breastfeeding in the United States.

   A. higher, lower

   B. lower, lower

   C. lower, higher

   D. higher, higher

14. The incidence of breastfeeding is likely to be lowest in which of these groups?

   A. Adolescents and new immigrants

   B. Women with advanced education

   C. Women with a supportive spouse or significant other

   D. Women who have successfully breastfed before

15. The highest percentage increase in incidence of breastfeeding in the United States from 1989 to 1992 was for what group?

   A. Adolescents

   B. Non-WIC participants

C. WIC participants
D. New immigrants

For questions 16 to 20, choose the best answer from the following key:

A. if responses 1, 2, and 3 are correct   **D. if response 4 is correct**
B. if responses 1 and 3 are correct   **E. if all are correct**
C. if responses 2 and 4 are correct

16. Barriers to breastfeeding include
    1. lack of support.
    2. too many rules.
    3. embarrassment.
    4. loss of freedom.

17. External factors that influence a marketing plan include
    1. political and legal issues in the marketplace.
    2. feelings that influence the mother's decision.
    3. economic conditions in the marketplace.
    4. conscious ambivalence toward breastfeeding by health-care workers.

18. Failure to determine the appropriate market for a product or service will result in
    1. additional markets for the product or service.
    2. an ineffective marketing plan.
    3. successful results for the growth of the product or service.
    4. lower consumer use of the product or service.

19. Making a marketing plan work requires
    1. planning.
    2. marketing research.
    3. sales.
    4. promotion.

20. Choosing the right mix of media to use in a marketing plan involves consideration of
    1. the targeted audience.
    2. budget constraints.
    3. the nature of the message.
    4. the mix used by the competitor.

History of Artificial Baby Milks

BREASTFEEDING/ARTIFICIAL BABY MILKS THROUGH THE AGES

Gatherer/Hunter Societies

Women acted as the breadwinners in the gatherer/hunter society, leading nomad existences. Menstruating and childbearing began later and stopped earlier, possibly because of marginal diets. Women breastfed for the first few years of the child's life. Rarely were children less than three to four years apart; women had five to six pregnancies in a lifetime.

Agricultural Societies

With the domestication of animals and the beginning of agricultural practices, the roles of women changed. Men were dependent on women for survival because of the need for their help in the fields. Women did more intense work, for longer periods, in this society than in the gathering/hunting society. Men pressured women to have more children to increase the "work force" and to feed babies foods other than breastmilk at an earlier age to facilitate weaning. Many gruels and artificial concoctions have been recorded as infant foods long before the twentieth century. Spouted feeding cups and feeding flasks have been found in the graves of infants dating back centuries before the Greek and Roman Empires.

Slavery

Initial thoughts were that it was easier and cheaper to buy slaves than lose labor while slaves bore and raised children. Slave owners awarded female slaves prizes for sterilization. Then theory changed and female slaves were encouraged to breed. Slave owners, however, only allowed slaves to breastfed for a limited time because breastfeeding prevented further breeding and decreased the amount of labor the slave provided.

Wet Nursing

Records trace shared suckling as far back as the pre-Christian era. Some reasons for wet nursing/shared suckling:

- As an act of female solidarity and cooperation
- Principally for reasons of social identification.

Noblewomen hired wet nurses because they were expected to delegate all physical labor. Their principle function was to provide heirs. Beliefs required breast-

Note: This synopsis is adapted from *The Politics of Breastfeeding* by Gabrielle Palmer (1988).

feeding women to abstain from sexual relations, and they knew that breastfeeding prevented pregnancy; wet nurses enabled noblewomen to conceive more often. Often only the eldest son was nursed by a noblewoman.

Sixteenth Century

Fashionable women wore corsets that caused damage to developing breasts, restricting and harming the nipples, preventing women from breastfeeding. Women with wealth bore many children but rarely breastfed. Mortality rates were high.

Pre-Industrial Revolution

Household units worked and lived in the same unit and breastfeeding fit into the system. Initially, inventors developed artificial baby milk for children who had no mother, and it originally consisted of: 10 cans milk/6 cans sugar/4 cans water/ 1 can oil and lime water.

Nineteenth Century

Industry developed techniques for condensing milk and marketed condensed milk as an infant food. Justus Von Liebig, "the father of modern nutrition," developed the "perfect infant food." It consisted of wheat flour, cow's milk, malt flour and bicarbonate of potash. Later, when creating a powder formula, he substituted pea flour for cow's milk. Doctors complained that babies where unable to digest Von Liebig's formula and doubted it was a counterpart to mother's milk (Palmer, 1988). Henri Nestlé sold 500,000 boxes a year of "farine lactee," continuing the development and use of breastmilk substitutes (Palmer, 1988).

AGRICULTURE AND MEDICINE ENDORSE ARTIFICIAL BABY MILKS

Agriculture played a role in the development of artificial baby milk. With the development of agriculture and the domestication of animals, nonhuman milk and supplies of starchy foods were available for use. Women started to feed their infants these foods at an earlier age and discontinued breastfeeding earlier. The earlier cessation of breastfeeding aided in increasing the population to help with agricultural work.

Improvements in dairy farming led to surpluses of milk, prompting markets to search for new market outlets (i.e., breastmilk substitutes). The baby milk market developed in the late nineteenth and early twentieth centuries through a mutual attraction of the manufacturers and the doctors, building on centuries of maternal practices of supplementing breastfeeding with other foods. Doctors took over the job of overseeing the birth process, increasing hospital deliveries. Doctors insisted babies have an individual formula prescribed by a doctor who would adjust it every few weeks.

INDUSTRY AND LOBBYISTS SUSTAIN ACCEPTANCE OF ARTIFICIAL BABY MILKS

Industrialization and urbanization developed a need for artificial baby milks. Urban working women were forced to be away from their babies, thus establishing a need for alternatives to breastfeeding. Industry, using the surplus of milk, new methods of preservation, and the materials and production methods to develop feeding bottles and teats, marketed a new feeding method for infants. Mothers began buying commercial formulas, abandoning frequent doctor visits for individualized formula. For supposed nutritional reasons, doctors objected to commercial formula. Realizing that a conflict with the medical profession was not advantageous, the formula manufactures joined forces with the doctors. The manufacturers marketed the formula without directions, with the label stating "consult your doctor for instructions," which economically benefitted both manufacturers and doctors.

EXPLOSION OF RESEARCH INTO INDIVIDUAL AND SOCIETAL BENEFITS FROM BREASTFEEDING

The health benefits of breastfeeding became evident when, in a 1910 Boston study, bottle-fed babies were found to be six times more likely to die than those who were breastfed. In 1911, a study in eight U.S. cities provided a sixfold risk of mortality in low-income families and a fourfold risk of mortality in high-income families who did not breastfeed. Over the remainder of the century, an explosion of research has shown the maternal and infant health benefits of breastfeeding. These benefits are the subject of Chapter 2 in this module.

FEEDING OF ARTIFICIAL BABY MILKS BECOMES THE NORM IN THE UNITED STATES

Social and behavioral changes follow several phases. The first phase is often called the traditional phase where high prevalence and duration of a change occurs after early promotional efforts. This is followed by a transformation phase in which prevalence and duration becomes shorter. Finally, a resurgence phase occurs with rising prevalence and duration. Different population groups arrive at each of these phases at different times. The lead social group is usually the urban elite, who are more educated and wealthy. The next group to respond is the middle class, with the rural poor being the most resistant to change and the last to embrace a new or different social behavior. The behavior of the urban middle class, urban poor, and rural poor are thus imitators of the urban elite, who are viewed as leading social and behavioral change and whose practices permeate to other groups. The abandonment or curtailment of breastfeeding has been viewed as a necessity forced on women by industrialization, employment of woman outside the family, and the breakdown of a supportive family structure, which, in short, is a result of socioeconomic change as each group passes from its traditional lifestyle. Many believe that changes in feeding behavior are a result of the pressures of changing lifestyles and the disappearance of traditional support systems.

Breastfeeding rates in the United States hit an all time low in 1973 with 26% of new mothers choosing it as the method to use. The baby-boomer population, whose current ages are between 29 and 50 years, now make up 40% of the adult population, with an estimated 75 million adults in the United States. Small, nuclear families replaced the extended, multigenerational families of the past. Geographic mobility has contributed to the disappearance of traditional support systems for families. This has resulted in a lack of available and/or knowledgeable female relatives to provide breastfeeding guidance.

Breastfeeding is a learned behavior that prior to this century in the United States had been taught informally by women who openly breastfed. The baby-boomer generation has been raised as a bottle-feeding culture, having themselves been fed by bottle and artificial baby milk. This is a generation with a high level of education that has been exposed since infancy to books, films, and other media that portray bottle feeding as the method of feeding babies and who have rarely seen women breastfeed in public. This population has seen breastfeeding as shameful and bottle feeding as normal and a source of pride. Breastfeeding mothers usually hide in public to breastfeed or cover up their infants with shawls. This generation has reacted publicly to breastfeeding in a negative manner to the point that laws have been required to ensure women the right to breastfeed in public. Although breastfeeding has been encouraged of late to the pregnant women of this generation, it has been seen as a question of choice and the feeding of artificial baby milk has been presented as just as good so that women do not feel guilty. The secular humanistic concept of tolerance has pervaded the infant feeding choice—it is not acceptable to view breastfeeding as the right way to feed a baby and bottle feeding artificial baby milk the wrong way to feed.

The attitude of health-care providers has been one of conscious ambivalence toward the infant-feeding decision. Educational curriculums are glaringly weak in the area of lactation management and have been slow to incorporate the vast arena of research regarding the superiority of breastfeeding. "I was raised on formula and I am all right" was a commonly heard phrase in the past decade. Ethical practices that would be taboo in many other areas of health care are condoned without question when professionals accept free gifts, honorariums, architectural planning services, gifts for patients, etc., from artificial baby milk manufacturers. Major health-care organizations that represent the very professionals who claim to promote breastfeeding accept extremely large gratuities for research and professional development from artificial baby milk manufacturers.

Only when a group reaches a stage of affluence or a degree of adaptation to the new lifestyle does a new behavior become easier to practice. Just as the urban elite led the movement to the use of bottles to provide artificial baby milk, they now lead the way back to breastfeeding. Rates of breastfeeding hit bottom, began rising, hit the transformation stage where they decreased slightly, and now have begun to rise again. The trickle down of behavioral change from the urban elite to the rural poor is most evident when one looks at the recent improvements in incidence data and duration of breastfeeding in the Special Supplemental Nutrition Program for Women, Infants, and Children (WIC) program. Measures that make it possible for women to breastfeed where otherwise outside pressures would have mitigated against the practice are being implemented and are successfully impacting duration rates.

RECOGNITION BY MEDICAL SOCIETIES AND GOVERNMENT THAT NORMS MUST CHANGE

1919: International Labour Organization (ILO) Convention No. 3

1952: International Labour Organization Convention No. 103. These conventions set standards to protect women in commerce and industry to include 12 weeks maternity leave (6 weeks before and after birth) to include cash benefits of at least 66% of previous earnings; two half-hour breaks during each workday to breastfeed and prohibition of dismissal during maternity leave (WABA, 1993).

1956: La Leche League International founded.

1977: Infant Formula Action Coalition (INFACT) coordinates Nestlé boycott.

1980: Infant Formula Act of 1980. Legislation drafted setting nutrient standards for infant formula. The formula companies opposed some regulations proposed and the American Medical Association (AMA) supported the formula companies; thus, the specifics of quality control were left up to the manufacturers.

1981: United States casts lone opposing vote to the World Health Organization (WHO) International Code of Marketing of Breast-milk Substitutes. The Code was adopted by 118 countries with three abstentions.

1981: Healthy Mothers, Healthy Babies Coalition formed.

1982: The U.S. Food and Drug Administration (FDA) was still drafting formula regulations, with the Reagan administration encouraging the FDA to weaken restrictions. The FDA finally published quality-control regulations for formula. These regulations were a compromise between the original draft and the formula companies' interest (Palmer, 1988).

1980–1990: Major health organizations published position papers supporting breastfeeding.

1984: U.S. Surgeon General's Workshop on Breastfeeding and Human Lactation held in Rochester, New York, and report published.

1984: Nestlé boycott ends.

1985: Follow-up report published from Surgeon General's Workshop on Breastfeeding and Human Lactation.

1987: European Strategy for Breastfeeding Promotion published.

1987: Center for Breastfeeding Information begun by La Leche League International.

1988: Nestlé boycott reinstated.

1989: WHO and United Nations Children's Fund (UNICEF) publish *Promoting and Supporting Breastfeeding: The Special Role of Maternity Services.*

1990: The Innocenti Declaration adopted at WHO/UNICEF meeting in Italy (August).

1990: Convention on the Rights of the Child (September).

1990: Breastfeeding Promotion Consortium formed.

1991:   Second follow-up report published on U.S. Surgeon General's Workshops on Breastfeeding and Human Lactation.

1992:   Breastfeeding Promotion Act signed (House of Representatives Bill 4322 and Senate Bill 2374), which allows the solicitation of private and public funds by USDA to mount a national media campaign promoting breast-feeding.

1992:   World Declaration and Plan of Action for Nutrition developed at the International Conference on Nutrition.

1994:   WHO reaffirms the Code of Marketing of Breast-milk Substitutes. The United States votes in favor of the code, reversing the position it took in 1981.

1994:   U.S. Department of Agriculture (USDA) issues final rule that requires the development of general standards to measure that Special Supplemental Nutrition Program for Women, Infants and Children (WIC) adequately supports and promotes breastfeeding.

1994:   Reauthorization of WIC program. Increases in federal dollars for breastfeeding from $8 million to $22 million, for an estimated $21.00 per participant.

1995:   FDA awarded a contract to Life Sciences Research Office of the Federation of American Societies for Experimental Biology to review the current nutrient requirements for infant formulas.

The Influence of Cultural Mores
on Breastfeeding

REEXAMINING WOMEN'S LIBERTIES AS DETERMINANTS OF BREASTFEEDING

Differences in social and cultural conditions exist within and outside communities and continents. Categorical groupings of breastfeeding behaviors by geographical locale leads to an oversimplification of the issues surrounding childbirth and breastfeeding. Vanessa Maher, in her book, *The Anthropology of Breastfeeding—Natural Law or Social Construct* (1992), questions how strict controls, which are mediated by the political and symbolic systems, on women's sexuality, reproductive capacities, and social relationships affect the practice of breastfeeding. She questions the medical model of viewing breastfeeding solely as a nutritional practice to nourish and prevent infection and disease. In her field experience in several developing countries, she has made observations about male–female relationships in cultures where adult male privileges are disproportionate, leading to what she terms gender inequality. Maher suggests that in such cultures breastfeeding as a solely womanly art has in fact led many impoverished women who already bear the burden of care-taking roles, domestic tasks, and agricultural duties to expend physical resources without monetary reward, contributing to high morbidity and low life expectancy for themselves. Thus for women in these populations, artificial baby milks give the women freedoms and reasons to require money of the more dominant gender—their male partners.

Sheila Kitzinger devotes a chapter in her book, *The Experience of Breastfeeding* (1987), to discussing the case for artificial feeding—primarily that, for whatever reason, it is the mother's choice. She states that because in many industrialized countries pregnancy and birth have been taken over by large institutions and modern technology, women may desire to reclaim their bodies, to include their breasts, and the decision to use them to feed the baby or not. To not impose guilt on the mother has been so overemphasized to health-care professionals that prominent speakers now remind professionals that giving the mother all the facts leads to an informed choice and not guilt regarding the infant feeding choice.

Socially determined attitudes and practices toward breastfeeding in most cultures contribute to the promotion, encouragement, and support of breastfeeding or the lack of those attributes. A wide range of beliefs, customs, and laws determines these attitudes and practices: Some cultures believe in milk kinship and women nurse babies other than their own to:

- Create family bonds to prevent marriages.
- Strengthen tribal unity.
- Promote alliances and make peace with enemy tribes.
- Demonstrate confidence between trading partners.

Other cultures believe in "bad milk." The belief that milk is bad and can harm the baby if the mother is hot, tired, angry, fatigued, pregnant, sleeping, unhappy, hungry, cold, or ill permeates some cultures. Some cultures believe semen in the body will spoil the milk and have postpartum taboos that prevent sexual intercourse while breastfeeding. Other cultures believe the qualities and defects of the woman who suckles a child pass on to the child through her milk.

BREASTFEEDING AROUND THE GLOBE

The following is a synopsis of information on breastfeeding practices around the world. It is by no means exhaustive and is only meant to give the reader a picture of historical and present-day practices in a few countries.

Africa

As a rule, women in most African countries practice long periods of breastfeeding and weaning. Some women use gruel as a supplement.

East Africa—The Masai of East Africa use breastfeeding as a means of making peace with other tribes. A breastfeeding woman from each tribe suckles the other's infant at the breast.

Tanzania (East Central Africa)—Women in the urban areas practice breastfeeding, bottle-feeding, and mixed feeding.

Middle East Africa—Women practice lengthy periods of breastfeeding as a rule. At one time, the Middle East Africans practiced milk kinship, using it to prevent marriages and promote alliances.

North Africa—Women practice lengthy periods of breastfeeding as a rule. Women will breastfeed in the company of other women. At one time, the North African practiced milk kinship, using it to prevent marriages and promote alliances.

Northern Tunisia—In this Muslim society, women are obligated to breastfeed their children for two years. The Northern Tunisian peasants believed that if a mother attempted to feed her child when she was tired and hot, the milk was "bad."

Northwest Mountains of Tunisia (Khroumirie)—Women breastfeed for approximately two years. It is the cultural belief that the flow of the mother's milk and the evidence that the mother's baby is thriving is a sign of "baraka," a life-sustaining force (Creyghton, 1992).

Sub-Sahara Africa—Breastfeeding in encouraged by kin and husbands. Women commonly breastfeed for two or more years. Most of the women do agricultural work.

Nigeria (West Africa)—Postpartum taboo prevented the mother from having sexual intercourse for two to three years. This period was frequently associated with the breastfeeding period. Present-day mothers still breastfeed for several months while utilizing supplements (Maher, 1992).

Guinea-Bissau—It is reported that mature breastmilk could turn bad in case of mother's sickness or adultery. Milk can be diagnosed as bad by putting an ant into it to observe if it dies (Gunnlaugsson & Einarsd'ottr, 1993).

Asia

The major problems identified in the Asia/Near East regions by the NGO Committee on UNICEF (Working Group on Nutrition) are as follows (Baumslag & Putney, 1989):

- *The Triple Nipple Syndrome*—This describes the shift from exclusive breastfeeding to mixed breast and bottle feeding with early supplementation.
- *Discarding Colostrum and the Use of Prelacteal Feeds*—Beliefs that colostrum is dirty and harmful are prevalent and have led to the practice of discarding colostrum and replacing it with clarified butter, dates, olive oil, honey, mashed banana, powdered milk, and formula.
- *Bottling the Breast*—This is when the concepts and practices related to bottle feeding are carried over to the process of breastfeeding. Examples include cleaning of the maternal nipples, feeding on a schedule, discarding the breastmilk if not the correct color, etc.

Central Asia

Nepal—In Mithila, the people feed children goat's milk to counteract any negative qualities of the mother. The women in the village of Salme in rural Nepal practice breastfeeding on demand and opportunity feeding. The village inhabitants are the Tamang, non-monastic Buddhists, who take the infants to work with them, and the Kami, Hindus, who do less work outside the home (Maher, 1992).

East Asia

Philippines—The women in the urban areas practice breastfeeding, bottle feeding, and mixed feeding. Earlier Filipinos believed in the idea of "bad milk" (Maher, 1992). Incidence and duration of breastfeeding have declined since 1973 particularly in urban, better-educated and higher income groups (Williamson, 1990). The National Movement for Promotion of Breastfeeding is working to improve hospital practices and implement a five-year plan. An alternative childcare service (Arugaan), which has been organized by and for women, provides wet nursing. Child-care centers are managed by breastfeeding mothers who nurse their own babies and others' babies (WABA, 1993).

Southwestern Asia

Iran—The Shi'ite Islamic in Iran believed the milk belonged to the husband. They also believed in milk kinship and prohibited intermarriage within this kinship. The Islamics introduced formula milk into the culture in the late 1940s. This led to the end of milk kinship in the middle and upper class who could afford to buy formula. Milk kinship is no longer a practiced belief. They use a few wet nurses but are very selective because they believe the qualities and defects of a woman pass to the child through the breastmilk (Khatib-Chahidi, 1992).

Iraq—In Baganda, infants of 1 year of age wean from the breast and the parents send them to the paternal grandmothers, who raise them (Maher, 1992).

Saudi Arabia—In this Muslim society, women are obligated to breastfeed their husbands' children for two years. However, from the 1950s through the 1970s, the elite began bottle feeding their infants; they have since returned to breastfeeding (Maher, 1992).

Israel—Breastfeeding practices differ among the two cultures in this country, with approximately 84% of the Jewish mothers breastfeeding for three months and 94.4% of the Arab mothers breastfeeding for five months (Heldenberg, Tenenbaum, & Weizer, 1993). In a study of the continuation of breastfeeding in an Israeli population, 40.3% of 633 mothers who initiated breastfeeding did so for three months. Orthodox religious belief was the most significant factor associated with long duration: 12.7% breastfed for 12 months (Birenbaum et al., 1993).

Negeu Bedouin Arabs of Israel—A ten-year, multidisciplinary research project to learn about the relationship between infant feeding, growth, and morbidity in this culture as it moves from seminomadism to urbanization has been reported recently (Hundt & Forman, 1993). This work used ethnographic data and merged epidemiology and anthropology in reporting the results. The reader is referred to this publication for information on the duration of exclusive breastfeeding during the traditional 40-day rest period in this population. This work is multifaceted and beyond the scope of this book but lends interesting insights into culture-specific practices and how they are studied.

Lebanon—In Beirut, the people believed in the concept of "bad milk." They had several beliefs about how milk could harm the infant:

- If the woman was angry or tired, the breastmilk would be hot and could harm the infant.
- If the woman was pregnant, the milk was poisonous.
- If the woman was lazy, the milk was considered "the milk of laziness" or "dead milk" (Maher, 1992).

Northeast Asia

Korea—A study of health-related behaviors in South Korea reported a 75.3% mean prevalence of breastfeeding in the urban area and an 81.1% prevalence in the rural area. Higher rates of breastfeeding were associated with an older maternal age and lower educational level (Chung et al., 1992–93).

Southern Asia

India—Hindus do not recognize milk ties in their laws, yet the wet nurse held hereditary status of "kinship by milk" (Panter-Brick, 1992). A study of women of high economic status and higher education levels in Jaykay Nagar, Kota India, showed that 51.7% of the women use prelacteal feeds of honey, 68.3% delayed the initiation of breastfeeding for more than 24 hours, 53% discarded the colostrum, and 83% introduced bottle feeding within the baby's first month of life (Singhania, Kabra, & Bansal, 1990). Most Indian women discard the colostrum, though the rural mothers are less likely to follow this practice (Subbulakshmi, Udipi, & Nirmalamma, 1990). Some construction sites are providing mobile creches for women working at them (WABA, 1993).

Southeastern Asia—Women practice lengthy periods of breastfeeding as a rule, using rice and water as a supplement (Maher, 1992).

Indonesia—A 1983 survey revealed a 98% breastfeeding initiation rate, an increase over the previous decade (Joesoef, 1989).

Malaysia—Studies show that 61% of the women breastfeed. The Malaysia Code of Ethics for Infant Formula Products was established to encourage an increase in this rate (Chia, 1992).

Thailand—Bangkok-Siriraj Hospital has a creche for infants up to 18 months old so that staff can breastfeed their babies at work (WABA, 1993).

Europe

The countries in Europe have practiced a variety of infant feeding techniques such as wet nursing, bottle feeding and other practices. Some areas and religions believe in milk-kinship.

Greece (Republic of Southeast Europe)—Greek women believe breastfeeding and weaning determines the confines of the self and its relationship to society. They also believe others who envy them may interfere with the weaning process and that a mother may cast an "evil eye" on others if she feels overtaxed by excessive breastfeeding. In Northern Greece, breastfeeding was considered the means by which mother and child pass from a "symbiotic relationship to their reciprocal definition as separate persons" (Maher, 1992).

Italy (South Europe)—Breastfeeding is considered natural and a cultural obligation and conviction. The mothers are generally great supporters of breastfeeding. Husbands encourage breastfeeding by helping with housework the first few weeks after delivery. Hospitals and local pediatricians tended to discourage breastfeeding in the late 1970s and 1980s with practices that encouraged separation, supplementation, feeding schedules, and disinfectant applied to the breast.

Italian law allows women to arrive late for work, to leave early, and to take up to two hours a day for breastfeeding. However, few women use this law for fear of the resentment of employers and colleagues.

In Turin, the ratio for feeding methods are 39% breastfeeding, 36% bottle feeding, and 22% mixed feeding. The hospitals in Turin practice separation of mother and child. In recent studies, doctors, husbands, and friends advised women not to breastfeed or to stop breastfeeding for fear of eyesight damage, possible malformation of the breast, illness, tiredness, or mishaps (Balsamo et al., 1992).

Switzerland—Incidence of breastfeeding is reported to be high even in a population of ill newborns, in which 50% of the women exclusively breastfeed and 25% partially breastfeed (Hunkeler et al., 1994).

United Kingdom—Over the last 100 years, bottle feeding has become the norm, a trend led by the United States, with only 26% of the women here breastfeeding for four months in 1980. Recent trends are working to encourage breastfeeding and reverse the bottle-feeding trend (Maher, 1992).

Scandinavia

In the 1970s and 1980s, breastfeeding duration increased dramatically, largely because of the availability of problem-based information material, rapid growth of mother-to-mother support groups in Sweden and Norway, more experienced health workers, prolonged maternity leaves, changes in maternity ward practices, low profiles of infant formula companies, the feminist movement's positive attitude toward breastfeeding, and a relaxed attitude toward breast exposure (Helsing, 1989).

Sweden—Breastfeeding has greatly increased in prevalence and in duration in the last decade (Larsson, Ogaard, & Lindsten, 1993).

Norway—The longest duration of breastfeeding is reported for Sami children. Maternity leave is 18 weeks (Larsson, Ogaard, & Lindsten, 1993).

Iceland—From 1600 to 1900, infants were fed cow's milk, cream, and chewed fish diluted with the former, and women rarely breastfed (Hastrup, 1992). Fertility was high during this time but so was infant mortality (300 per 1,000). Only 2 or 3 of the 12 to 15 children born to a married couple would reach adulthood. One traveling physician in the mid-eighteenth century attributed the high infant mortality rate to be, in part, because the mothers did not breastfeed (Hastrup, 1992).

Oceania

New Guinea—The trend was to breastfeed for long periods without the use of transitional or weaning foods. They believed that breastfeeding provided imagery for religious beliefs. Traditionally the men in the society decided who breastfed whom and for how long. However, the trend is changing because of concern that husbands may leave if the mother pays too much attention to the infant. They are also bottle feeding in an attempt to make the husbands responsible for some parenting by having to purchase formula. Some women formula feed in a desire to share the parental role with others (husbands, grandparents). Postpartum taboos also existed preventing the mother from having sexual intercourse for two to three years. This period was frequently associated with the breastfeeding period (Maher, 1992). Beginning in 1977, infant formula, bottles, and nipples can only be obtained by prescription (Baumslag & Putney, 1989).

Australia—Australia has an active group of professionals and lay persons promoting and supporting breastfeeding. The Nursing Mothers' Association of Australia (NMAA) publishes *Breastfeeding Review*, which is available twice per year by subscription. Australia's national affiliate of the International Lactation Consultant Association (ILCA) is the Australian Lactation Consultant Association (ALCA).

Latin America

Brazil—The incidence of breastfeeding declined during the 1960s and 1970s and now there is a campaign within the country to change this trend (Baumslag & Putney, 1989). This campaign has been in effect since 1981 and per a 1984–85 survey, breastfeeding is initiated by 93% of new mothers (Monteiro et al., 1988).

Honduras—A significant increase in initiation and duration of breastfeeding was reported among Honduran women between 1981 and 1987. The PROALMA breastfeeding promotion program is believed to have had a profound effect on the breastfeeding behavior of women in this population (Popkin et al., 1991).

Mexico—A report from the 1986 National Health Survey found that 19.9% of Mexican infants were never breastfed and that 42.4% received breastmilk for three months or less (Gomez et al., 1990). "Maria Liberacion" is a group in Central Mexico that supports domestic workers in negotiating for better arrangements during and after pregnancy, including the ability to breastfeed while working (WABA, 1993).

Uruguay—In the public sector, women are allowed to work half-time in order to breastfeed during the first six months of their baby's life while receiving 100% of their salary (WABA, 1993).

North America

Canada—Breastfeeding rates vary widely in Canada with higher rates (80%) reported for Ontario and lower rates (50%) for Quebec. Mothers receive $50.00 a month for breastfeeding, if on government assistance, but less ($17.50) if formula feeding. In Alberta and British Columbia, mothers are routinely visited by a community nurse within 24 hours of discharge. The Canadian Institute of Child Health has multicultural information on breastfeeding available in 13 languages (Backas, 1996).

United States—Over the last 100 years, bottle feeding has become the norm. Recently various groups have been working to encourage breastfeeding and reverse the bottle-feeding trend.

Other than in this section, the descriptions of trends in infant feeding, positive and negative factors influencing breastfeeding, myths about breastfeeding, etc., found in this module pertain to the United States.

Important Factors in the Decision
to Breastfeed

In working to change from a formula to breastmilk culture, the many factors that may influence a mother's decision to breastfeed have been the subject of research for investigators of various disciplines. Social and health scientists have explored the infant-feeding decision-making process extensively. Socioeconomic status, level of self-esteem, educational level, age, social milieu, and ethnicity all influence a woman's infant feeding choice (Baranowski et al., 1983; Rassin et al., 1984, 1993). Newton's (1967) work shows us that the degree to which a woman is accepting of her biologic role as a female directly affects her "psychosexual behavior," which includes breastfeeding. Kocturk and Zetterstrom (1989) conclude, in their review of a variety of studies that looked at the reasons why women breastfeed, that in societies where women experience a high degree of repression, biological functions that otherwise are pleasurable, may be regarded as burdens.

The health-care provider can exert a positive influence on a mother's decision to breastfeed her infant. To be effective, however, it is crucial that they consider the intricate nature of a good support network. The goals should be to educate women in all aspects of normal lactation and to enable them to move toward becoming a successful nursing dyad (McNatt & Freston, 1992). We know that the culture, geographic location, and level of support should be among the factors considered when formulating a plan to help breastfeeding mothers.

Baranowski and his colleagues (1986) have explored a mother's ethnic background and the weight of influence family members have on her decision to breastfeed, her perception of her breastfeeding experience, and the length of time she will breastfeed her infant. African American, Hispanic, and Asian American mothers whose demographic profiles include more than 12 years of formal education and being married, cite their husband or male partner as the most important support person after the decision to breastfeed is made. Those in the health-care setting should target new fathers, whenever possible, by including them in prenatal breastfeeding classes and contact sessions.

PRENATAL EDUCATION

 As breastfeeding became less acceptable as the obvious method of feeding by mothers, fewer girls grew up seeing or hearing about successful breastfeeding. The present generation of women represent these girls; therefore, it is the responsibility of health-care workers and breastfeeding advocates to educate women and their families about the benefits of and approaches to successful breastfeeding. Attendance at prenatal education programs favorably affects feeding practices (although it is not known whether those who attend prenatal classes are those already motivated to breastfeed), increasing not only the number of women who initiate breastfeeding, but also its duration (Brogan & Fox, 1984; Giugliani et al., 1994; Kistin et al., 1990; Matich & Sims, 1992). Physicians who provide obstetrical care should provide educational materials on breastfeeding, information on lactation support groups, and sources for breast pumps because this may influence the infant-feeding decision (Starbird, 1991; Williams & Pan, 1994), although this has not been found to occur consistently (Giugliani et al., 1994). In one study, physicians were found to be the second most important determinant in the decision to formula feed (Novotny et al., 1994).

Kaplowitz and Olson (1983) concluded that once a woman decides how to feed her baby, she does not change her mind and that being knowledgeable about breastfeeding without having accompanying positive attitudes does not ensure that a woman will breastfeed. A positive attitude about breastfeeding was cited as the most important determinant of infant-feeding choice in a group of low-income women in the Southeast (Black et al., 1990); this includes the choice to breast- or bottle feed with a high correlation between a negative attitude toward breastfeeding and the choice to formula feed. Research shows women tend to decide to breastfeed either prior to conception or during pregnancy (Littman et al., 1994). Novotny et al. (1994) found 47% of feeding-method decisions are made prior to pregnancy, 25% after birth, with less than 15% of women choosing a method of feeding during each trimester of pregnancy. Women who formula feed tend to make up the 25% who select a feeding method after the infant is born.

Prenatal education concerning breastfeeding should target women in high school or early in pregnancy (Pascoe & Berger, 1985). Prenatal education may be provided by hospitals or clinics, private classes, support groups, and/or literature. The clients for each of these areas will vary greatly in culture, age, marital status, ethnicity, and education levels. The education material, therefore, needs to be designed to be culture-specific. Successful programs include education in a language and mode that the target population finds understandable and acceptable. It should address fears and concerns about breastfeeding in order to create a positive attitude toward breastfeeding. Educational material should include the benefits of breastfeeding for the infant and the mother but emphasize the techniques necessary to be successful. Material and programs should include information on pumping, storing, and collecting milk.

PERCEPTION OF BENEFITS

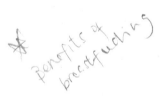

"Breastfeeding is an integral part of the reproductive process, the natural and ideal way of feeding the infant, and a unique biological and emotional basis for child development" (WHO, 1981). The many physical, emotional, and psychological benefits of breastfeeding are widely recognized in many sectors, but an individual mother's perception of these benefits will provide the greatest incentive for choosing breastfeeding.

By choosing breastfeeding, a mother is making an emotional commitment that lasts a lifetime. Breastfeeding is one way for a mother to fulfill her aspiration to give love to her baby. A special and long-term relationship between mother and baby is created that is not easily duplicated. Mothers who have breastfed previous children will cite the private time they experience with their infants during nursing as something only a mother can enjoy with her child. The hormones oxytocin and prolactin induce a state of relaxation, warmth, and love.

For some mothers, convenience is often perceived as an advantage of breastfeeding. Human milk is always ready in the correct amount, at the right temperature.

Breastfeeding gives a mother more time to enjoy her baby because she does not need to spend time focusing on bottles and their preparation. She is able to respond to her infant's signals immediately, resulting in less anxiety for baby and mother. When mothers learn to read their infants' cues and respond to them, infants can organize their behavior and learn to trust themselves and others.

Many women know that breastfeeding offers the infant protection from infection, fewer allergies, optimum nutrition (refer to Chapter 2 in this module), and, in general, increased good health. Most breastfeeding mothers discuss their feelings about the benefits with pride and conviction that they are giving their infants the best start in life. The mother also benefits physically from breastfeeding. Breastfeeding aids in postpartum weight loss, it prolongs postpartum amenorrhea, and it exerts a protective effect against premenopausal breast cancer. The family also benefits from the mother who breastfeeds. The economical advantage breastfeeding provides is seen by many mothers as a direct benefit for all the family members because less of the household resource pool is diverted to infant feeding. Unfortunately, many of these benefits are perceived as barriers for some women and are discussed in the Factors that Negatively Influence the Decision to Breastfeed section in this chapter.

SOCIODEMOGRAPHIC FACTORS

Many studies conducted in the United States and abroad aid in detecting which mothers are most likely to breastfeed. A variety of demographics seem to influence breastfeeding initiation and duration, both positively and negatively. Though the incidence of breastfeeding appears to be steadily increasing throughout the United States (see Figure 1A–1), some regions of the country have a higher prevalence than other regions. Mothers in the Mountain and Pacific regions continue to show a higher duration of breastfeeding (see Table 1A–1). Women in the Southeast region have the lowest breastfeeding-initiation rate (Martinez & Nalezienski, 1981; Ryan et al., 1991b).

Figure 1A–1

Breastfeeding initiation trends for all groups— 1988 to 1995.

Source: Adapted from *Connections MCHB*, 1993, p. 2, and Ross Laboratories from Mothers' Survey, 1993–95. Used with permission of Ross Products Division, Abbott Laboratories, Columbus, OH 43216. © 1993, 1994, 1995 Ross Products Division, Abbott Laboratories.

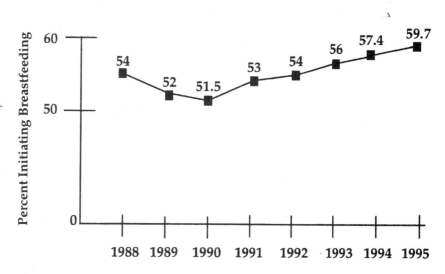

Table 1A-1 Percentage Breastfeeding Among All Infants at 5 to 6 Months of Age for Selected Demographics

	1986	1987	1988	1989	1990	1991	1992	1993
All Infants	23.1	21.8	21.1	19.6	19.0	19.7	20.4	20.6
Primiparous	19.8	18.8	18.4	16.6	16.2	17.0	18.2	18.9
Multiparous	26.8	25.2	24.2	22.7	21.8	22.0	21.9	21.6
Grade school	13.3	10.9	10.9	12.3	11.3	13.5	14.3	13.9
High school	16.6	15.7	14.7	13.4	12.8	13.2	13.8	14.2
No college	16.4	15.5	14.6	13.4	12.7	13.2	13.8	14.2
College	35.4	33.3	33.0	31.1	30.0	29.8	30.7	30.6
Employed full time	11.6	11.3	11.3	10.2	10.5	11.6	12.8	13.4
Employed part time	26.6	24.3	23.9	23.0	22.5	23.3	24.1	23.8
Total employed	17.0	15.9	15.8	14.8	14.7	15.8	16.7	17.1
Not employed	27.1	26.0	24.9	23.1	22.3	22.6	23.1	23.2
Less than $10,000	9.2	8.8	8.7	8.9	8.3	8.5	9.4	10.3
$10,000–$14,999	18.7	16.8	14.8	15.0	13.3	13.9	15.0	15.5
$15,000–$24,999	25.6	23.8	23.1	20.4	19.0	19.3	19.9	19.9
$25,000 +	31.4	29.6	29.0	27.6	27.1	27.4	28.3	27.9
Less than 20 years	7.4	7.5	6.7	6.2	6.3	6.5	6.8	7.5
20–24 years	16.8	15.5	14.4	12.7	12.1	12.4	13.4	13.9
25–29 years	27.1	25.6	24.5	22.9	21.2	21.4	22.3	22.6
30–34 years	35.6	33.0	33.5	31.4	30.0	29.3	29.8	29.4
35 + years	36.2	36.4	36.6	36.2	34.9	35.1	35.1	34.3
New England	25.9	24.5	23.2	20.3	21.8	21.3	21.5	21.3
Middle Atlantic	22.5	20.7	20.8	18.4	17.8	18.2	18.9	19.1
East North Central	21.2	20.0	18.7	18.1	17.4	18.0	18.9	18.7
West North Central	23.4	21.3	20.6	19.9	19.4	20.2	20.5	20.2
South Atlantic	18.1	17.3	16.3	14.8	15.0	15.7	16.7	17.4
East South Central	13.7	13.7	12.8	12.4	11.4	11.6	12.6	13.2
West South Central	16.7	16.9	16.2	14.7	13.9	15.2	15.6	15.7
Mountain	35.0	33.1	31.6	30.4	29.2	29.8	29.3	30.0
Pacific	34.2	31.2	31.0	28.7	27.5	27.8	29.4	29.3
Black	8.4	7.9	7.7	7.0	6.8	7.3	8.6	9.3
White	26.5	25.2	24.3	22.7	22.1	22.6	23.3	23.3
Hispanic	17.7	15.9	15.8	15.0	14.2	16.1	17.0	17.8

Note: Income for 1986–1988 is less than $7,000 and $7,000–$14,999.

Source: Used with permission of Ross Products Division, Abbott Laboratories, Columbus, OH 43216, from Mothers' Survey, © 1986–1993 Ross Products Division, Abbott Laboratories.

Parity

初産

Parity influences the incidence of breastfeeding. Women who have successfully breastfed their first child are 75% to 90% more likely to breastfeed the second child. However, if a mother is unsuccessful with the first child, she is only 22–24% likely to breastfeed her second child (Wade, 1994). Primiparous mothers show a stronger correlation between breastfeeding and education than multiparous women. Primiparous mothers account for the greatest rise in the proportion of infants ever breastfed (Becerra & Smith, 1990).

more than 1 child

Education/Marital Status/Income

Research has consistently showed a correlation between increased educational level and increased incidence of breastfeeding after 1965 in the United States. The 1989 Ross Mothers' Survey showed rapid increases in breastfeeding by women with less education (see Table 1A–2). Studies have not shown significant differences by education in African American or Hispanic groups but have in Anglo-European groups (Rassin et al., 1984). Marital status is also an important determinant of breastfeeding (Baranowski et al., 1983; Rassin et al., 1984, 1993; Wright et al., 1988). Low-income women have lower rates of breastfeeding in general (see Table 1A–3).

Employment

Employment does not seem to influence the breastfeeding-initiation rate (Littman et al., 1994). Yet, those mothers who do choose to breastfeed and are employed outside the home have a lower duration rate (see Table 1A-1) than those not employed outside the home (Martinez, Dodd, & Samartgedes, 1981; Meftuh, Tapsoba, & Lamounier, 1991). Lower duration rates for working women are attributed to lack of adequate familial, social, and professional support and insensitive employment environments (Becerra & Smith, 1990). Lack of support in the workplace and lack of time to pump may contribute to the lower duration rates among employed women.

Table 1A–2   Breastfeeding Rates by Educational Level

	At Birth		At 5 to 6 Months	
	WIC	Non-WIC	WIC	Non-WIC
No College	31.1%	52.5%	7.8%	18.4%
College	50.7%	74.6%	16.5%	33.9%

Source: Used with permission of Ross Products Division, Abbott Laboratories, Columbus, OH 43216, from Mothers' Survey, 1993, © 1993 Ross Products Division, Abbott Laboratories.

Table 1A–3   Breastfeeding Initiation and Duration Rates by Income Level

	In Hospital	At 5 to 6 Months
<10,000	37.5%	10.3%
10,000–14,999	48.8%	15.5%
15,000–24,999	56.2%	27.9%
25,000	68.6%	19.9%

Source: Used with permission of Ross Products Division, Abbott Laboratories, Columbus, OH 43216, from Mothers' Survey, 1993, © 1993 Ross Products Division, Abbott Laboratories.

Ethnicity

Rassin et al. (1984) were one of the first groups to report the importance of ethnicity on a mother's decision to breastfeed. They reported the incidence of breastfeeding to be lowest in low socioeconomic groups, especially in the African American population (see Table 1A–1). Mexican Americans also have a lower breastfeeding initiation rate and perceive breastfeeding as a physical inconvenience (Baranowski et al., 1986). Southeast Asians living in the United States tend to breastfeed at a much lower rate than they did while living in Southeast Asia and at a lower rate than Caucasians (Tuttle & Dewey, 1994). Rassin et al. (1993) studied the relationship of acculturation to the initiation of breastfeeding and found that women being assimilated into the United States are inhibited in the initiation of breastfeeding.

Sources of social support vary by ethnic group. Among African Americans the best friend has been found to be the most important influence, for Mexican Americans the mother's mother was most influential, and for Caucasians the male partner was most significant in the infant-feeding decision (Baranowski et al., 1983). Bryant (1982) also found that the husband was important only in the Caucasian population, with the mother's mother cited as important for Cuban and Puerto Rican women living in the United States. Bevan et al. (1984) reported the father to be influential in an urban WIC program of mixed ethnicity. Black et al. (1990) found the father of the infant to be important in the infant-feeding decision of Caucasian and African American women regardless of marital status. Littman et al. (1994) reported strong approval by the father was associated with a high incidence in a group of middle-income, Caucasian married women. Among predominantly Caucasian women planning to breastfeed, Freed et al. (1992) reported that the father of the baby was more likely to support the decision. In general, education and support efforts should be aimed at the person or persons who form the support network for mothers in a target population.

Maternal Age

Research shows a correlation between maternal age (see Table 1A–4) and breastfeeding incidence (Rassin et al., 1993). Breastfeeding initiation rates are lower among teenagers (Amador et al., 1992), with teenagers who were breastfed or those exposed to breastfeeding showing the highest incidence of breastfeeding among this age group (Lizarraga et al., 1992). Novotny et al. (1994) further conclude that women under 25 are least likely to breastfeed, although the rate of exclusive breastfeeding increases with maternal age. Older women are more likely to breastfeed their infants.

Table 1A–4   Breastfeeding Rates by Maternal Age

	At Birth		At 5 to 6 Months	
Maternal Age	WIC	Non-WIC	WIC	Non-WIC
Under 20 years	26.2%	40.8%	4.2%	10.9%
35 years and older	42.5%	71.5%	19.2%	39.9%

Source: Used with permission of Ross Products Division, Abbott Laboratories, Columbus, OH 43216, from Mothers' Survey, 1993, © 1993 Ross Products Division, Abbott Laboratories.

Many factors positively influence a mother's breastfeeding decision. However, there are also many factors that may negatively influence a mother's decision to breastfeed. These negative influences must be identified and understood in order to be overcome.

Initiation rates among WIC and non-WIC participants have shown increases since 1989 (see Table 1A–5). The percentage increase has been higher for WIC participants than for non-WIC participants.

Table 1A–5   Percentage of Women Who Breastfed in 1989 and 1992

	1989	1992[a]	Percentage point increase[b]	Percentage increase
WIC				
In hospital	34.8	38.9	4.1	11.8
One month	27.3	30.8	3.5	12.8
Three months	16.7	18.9	2.2	13.2
NON-WIC				
In hospital	62.9	66.1	3.2	5.1
One month	54.7	57.5	2.8	5.1
Three months	39.4	41.8	2.4	6.1

[a]Data are for the period October 1991 through September 1992

[b]All percentage point changes in breastfeeding rates for WIC mothers and non-WIC mothers between 1989 and 1992 were statistically significant at the 0.05 level.

Source: Used with permission of Ross Products Division, Abbott Laboratories, Columbus, OH 43216, from Mothers' Survey, 1989 to 1992, © 1989–1992 Ross Products Division, Abbott Laboratories.

Factors That Negatively Influence
the Decision to Breastfeed

In spite of the strong endorsement of breastfeeding by the American Academy of Pediatrics, the American Public Health Association, the American Dietetics Association, and the Office of the Surgeon General of the United States, negative attitudes and mythical ideas about breastfeeding abound. As the number of women breastfeeding increases, societal exposure to breastfeeding behavior will also increase; this might, in turn, facilitate a narrowing of the gap between real and perceived barriers to breastfeeding.

PERCEPTION OF BARRIERS

Much of what we have learned about barriers comes from group interviews by the Best Start Program and other research that identified "too many rules" as barriers (Bryant & Roy, 1990; Gabriel et al., 1986). A lack of confidence and insecurity on the part of the mother is a common factor that exerts a negative effect. She may feel that she will not have enough milk to adequately nourish her baby. She may question the quality of her milk (too thin, blue). Some women use artificial supplementation to cope with the fear of inadequate milk; this in turn creates a negative cycle of decreased milk production, confirming the fear. Inadequate information about the mechanics of lactation and breastfeeding management can also serve to undermine confidence. Some women feel that breastfeeding requires complicated or bothersome techniques that are difficult to learn; and even though they may feel that mother's milk is best for babies, choose artificial milk. Consistent information about frequency of feeding, the supply-and-demand nature of the lactation process, and neonatal behavior at the breast can break this cycle and begin to build and nurture confidence. In the early phase of breastfeeding, the infant's cueing system can be misinterpreted by the mother and other adult members that the baby is hungry. Lack of understanding concerning the normal mechanism of breastfeeding can prematurely end breastfeeding before it is well established.

Lacking breastfeeding role models in her immediate community, a mother may not see herself reflected in available promotional materials. She may feel breastfeeding is "not for" the specific group of which she feels herself a member (i.e., teen, low income, professional/employed). When a mother lacks confidence, it is then important to detect and explore her concerns and address them in a specific manner. She might conclude that her reality cannot include a breastfeeding relationship with her infant. Well-chosen, culture-sensitive materials can encourage a commitment to breastfeeding.

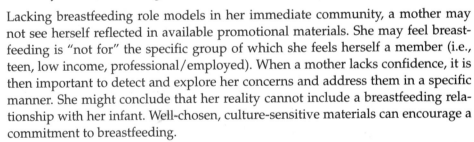

Mothers who worry about discouragement and lack of psychosocial support from family and friends are less likely to breastfeed. Anecdotes by others of their negative experiences with breastfeeding can interfere with a mother's resolve to choose and subsequently continue breastfeeding. Often, negative statements made by the husband, boyfriend, or the woman's mother can shake her confidence in her ability to breastfeed.

Table 1A–6   Why Aren't More Mothers Breastfeeding?—Cultural Factors

LIMITED ROLE MODELS

Today a generation of women in the United States have not breastfed and, therefore, are unable to support and advise new mothers on breastfeeding.

LOSS OF FREEDOM

Breastfeeding is often seen as incompatible with an active social life, and women fear it will prevent them from going to work, school, and social events.

"SPOILING" ISSUE

Many women do not breastfeed for fear that the infants will become spoiled and want to constantly be with their mother.

MEDIA INFLUENCE

The media portrays bottle feeding as the norm.

EMBARRASSMENT

Many women feel embarrassment when nursing in front of others. This is often because the breast is seen as a sexual object and women worry that breastfeeding in public will:

• arouse men
• make their husbands or boyfriends jealous
• make other women jealous
• look "gross" or "disgusting"

Many women also feel they would be embarrassed if their breasts leaked and others could see the stains on their clothing.

IMMIGRATION

New immigrants perceive formula feeding as a cultural norm and, in an effort to assimilate to a new culture, they formula feed. Also, they perceive the free distribution of formula through WIC as sponsoring and encouraging the use of formula. Advertising encourages the use of "new improved" products that lead the new immigrants to believe formula is better than breastmilk.

Source: Walker, M. (1992). Why aren't more mothers breastfeeding? *Childbirth Instr, Winter.* Used with permission.

These comments, or the lack of support from these individuals, are made out of jealousy, as a result of misinformation they have heard, and/or out of concern for the mother's well-being. The support of these individuals is crucial and educational material specifically addressed to key individuals in a mother-to-be's life will help educate them on the importance of and how to encourage breastfeeding. Formula material concerning breastfeeding often accentuates problems such as sore breasts and engorgement. Grandmothers were taught formula feeding was "best" and must be informed that "we" (health-care providers) were wrong and free them of guilt about their decisions (Frederickson, 1994).

Another common deterrent is the anticipated loss of freedom many women associate with breastfeeding an infant. "Our society has assumed that there is no valid intellectual stimulation to be had in the company of young children . . . in response new mothers panic to maintain their social and professional ties" (Lawrence, 1989). Breastfeeding is seen as incompatible with a "real life." Young mothers are concerned that breastfeeding will keep them from having time with their friends or interfere with school obligations. Mothers with established careers worry that the transition through new motherhood to the professional world cannot practically include breastfeeding. The undeniable mother–infant attachment that accompanies breastfeeding often does not accommodate return to pre-baby lifestyles. After the birth of her baby, a mother may move between feeling of oneness with and separation from the new baby. There is a natural and healthy psychological transition from oneness to separateness that each mother and baby must make.

The fear that a breastfed infant cannot be left with a sitter necessitates the availability of information on maintaining lactation even when mother and baby must be separated. Lack of support in the workplace is evidenced by the general climate at most jobsites (i.e., no pumping provisions, threat of loss of seniority, no on-site child care, inflexible leave policies, etc.). There is a trend in some corporate settings toward sanction and encouragement of family-oriented policies to include company-sponsored childbirth education and lactation programs.

Embarrassment is often a result of the preoccupation of the breast as an object of sexual focus rather than consideration of the biologic tool of nurturing babies. Women may worry that breastfeeding their baby will make husbands or boyfriends jealous, be immodest, or look "weird or disgusting." Fear of exposing or touching the breast may discourage a mother. A woman may feel uncomfortable nursing in front of others, but resent having to hide to feed her infant. Counseling and educational material on discrete nursing practices may enable women to feel more comfortable when nursing in front of others. The unpredictable nature of the milk ejection reflex in the early weeks of breastfeeding can be a source of embarrassment. With proper counseling about breast pads, good bras, and logistical techniques, this source of embarrassment can be reduced.

Women are often concerned that they must follow special dietary and health practices to breastfeed. They choose not to breastfeed out of fear of being unable or unwilling to change present dietary and health practices. They are concerned that they must stop all smoking and drinking of alcohol, drink more milk, follow special diets, sleep more, and remain relaxed. Counseling should alleviate these concerns with realistic advice on each issue that concerns the individual woman.

The issue of unconscious ambivalence can interfere with successful initiation and establishment of breastfeeding. Many women face conflicting desires; moving between the need to nurture their infants and the societal pressure to continue life as if childless. Lawrence (1989) noted that it has been generally accepted by proponents of breastfeeding that one of the major reasons to breastfeed is to provide that special relationship and closeness that accompanies nursing; although we know this to be true, this very relationship remains, for many, a major contraindication to breastfeeding.

Presenting breastfeeding as the superior choice in infant feeding is often approached with ambivalence by health-care professionals who have contact with women in the childbearing years. These women are formulating their ideas about breastfeeding; this attitude of ambivalence leaves the impression that on the whole there is no compelling reason to select breastfeeding over artificial feeding. According to Lawrence (1989), the worry over creating a feeling of guilt in the

Table 1A-7   Why Aren't More Mothers Breastfeeding?—Personal Factors

LACK OF CONFIDENCE

Because of misunderstandings or a lack of understanding of the mechanics of breastmilk production, many women lack confidence in their ability to produce an adequate quality or quantity of breastmilk. Also, many women fear that breastfeeding requires techniques that are difficult to learn.

LACK OF POSITIVE MODELS

For many women, the experience of watching an infant go to breast is foreign. No one they know is breastfeeding and they do not want to be different from their friends or relatives; this lack of role models leads to a decision to formula feed.

LACK OF SUPPORT (INFLUENCE OF FAMILY AND FRIENDS)

Family and friends with negative feelings about breastfeeding can greatly influence an expectant mother's decision on whether or not to breastfeed.

CONCERN ABOUT DIETARY AND HEALTH PRACTICES

Many women fear that breastfeeding will require them to change their dietary and/or health practices, such as:

- giving up smoking
- giving up drinking alcoholic beverages
- drinking enough milk
- following special dietary guidelines (e.g., no junk food, no spicy food)
- getting enough sleep
- relaxing

Source: Walker, M. (1992). Why aren't more mothers breastfeeding? *Childbirth Instr, Winter.* Used with permission.

mother who does not choose breastfeeding has led to an ambivalent attitude on the part of clinicians regarding infant-feeding discussions. As a result, many mothers are not provided the information necessary to make an informed choice.

COMMUNITY MYTHS

Many myths influence a woman's decision to breastfeed, the way a mother breastfeeds, and when a mother weans an infant. Myths can cause women to doubt their ability to breastfeed and create a lack of confidence when they do not hold true. The supporting literature for the following myths is described in more detail in subsequent modules of this series. The following compilation of myths are summarized from articles by Auerbach (1990b), Bernshaw (1992), and the *Circle of Caring* newsletter (Ameda Egnell, 1991).

Breastfeeding is natural; there is no need to learn about it.   Many women are told that breastfeeding is natural and that there is no need to learn about it. It is

Table 1A–8   Why Aren't More Mothers Breastfeeding?—Health-Care
System Factors

PROFESSIONAL NEUTRALITY

Many professionals allow parents to believe that bottle feeding and breastfeeding offer equal benefits.

BIRTH SETTING BARRIERS

Many health-care facilities are set up in such a manner as to make breastfeeding not only difficult but, at times, almost impossible.

LACK OF PRACTICAL ASSISTANCE

Many health-care workers have never been educated on breastfeeding techniques and, therefore, are unable to assist new mothers.

WIC DISTRIBUTION OF FORMULA

Many women see WIC distribution of formula as sponsoring and encouraging the use of formula.

LIMITED FOLLOW-UP CARE

With the lack of health-care workers educated in breastfeeding management, there is often no one to assist mothers with breastfeeding after they are discharged from the hospital.

Source: Walker, M. (1992). Why aren't more mothers breastfeeding? *Childbirth Instr, Winter.* Used with permission.

true that breastfeeding is natural, but not intuitive. In the present culture of most developed countries, there are few breastfeeding examples available and a generation lacks breastfeeding experience. Breastfeeding educational classes offer beneficial information to women who plan to breastfeed.

Formula is as good as breastmilk.   In a community that has formula fed for a generation, the myth that formula is as good as breastmilk developed. This is a definite myth. If formula was as good as breastmilk, why would formula companies try to develop formulas that are "closest to mother's milk"? Formula-fed infants have a higher morbidity and mortality rate. Formulas have the potential to be and are often adulterated during manufacturing. This places the baby at risk. Human milk contains live immune cells that protect the infant and growth factors that aid in normal growth, maturation, and functioning of the gastrointestinal tract. Formula does not have immune cells and growth factors.

Working women cannot continue to breastfeed after returning to work.   With more women working away from the home, returning to work while breastfeeding is a concern. One myth is that women cannot breastfeed when they return to work. This is untrue; once the milk is established a mother can express her milk when away from the infant. Mothers also report that breastfeeding helps them to feel they have not lost the special closeness they felt with their infants prior to returning to work. These mothers need adequate information, planning, and support for successful breastfeeding when returning to work.

Fair-skinned women are more susceptible to experiencing sore nipples.   Especially fair-skinned women are not predisposed to nipple tenderness, pain, and trauma. This myth can discourage many women from breastfeeding. Research has shown this myth has no basis. Scandinavian women do not report a higher rate of nipple soreness than other women. African American mothers are just as likely to experience nipple soreness as anyone else. Correct positioning at the breast is the critical factor in avoiding sore nipples.

Is the breast empty after breastfeeding or expressing milk?   Women often believe that the breast empties during or after breastfeeding. In actuality, sucking stimulates the breast to release the stored milk and to begin producing additional milk. Only bottles empty as the infant feeds; the lactating breast is never empty.

The more the baby nurses, the more milk is produced.   A baby who is not positioned correctly at the breast will "nurse" for longer periods of time (30–60 minutes) at each feeding, may cause nipple soreness, may fall asleep while nursing, will be unsatisfied after such a long "nursing" time, and the mother will have an inadequate supply of milk. A baby who is correctly latched on will stimulate the milk ejection reflex effectively. In turn, the baby will obtain the calorie-rich hind milk. A baby may want to feed for longer periods of time (10–30 minutes) or may have closeness and sucking needs independent of nutrition. Proper positioning and latching on is essential for effective feeding and for the mother's comfort.

Pain is normal during the early days/weeks of breastfeeding.   As Newton (1971) points out, key survival responses are pleasurable, thereby increasing the likelihood that they will by repeated. It is the same with breastfeeding; it should be a pleasurable and relaxing experience. If it hurts, there is something wrong, most likely positioning.

A mother who wishes to breastfeed should "toughen" her nipples.   Studies have shown that brisk rubbing or twisting of the nipple does little to prevent soreness and actually increases soreness. Furthermore, rubbing with a towel removes protective oils and cells. This causes abrasion and nipple tenderness and the skin to be more prone to infection. Also, "toughening" of the nipple causes it to desensitize and become less responsive, reducing its ability to function.

Engorgement is normal.   Severe engorgement is not physiologic and may prevent the infant from grasping the nipple and impedes the release of milk. Frequent, effective nursing can prevent engorgement. Transient breast fullness is experienced by nearly all nursing women during times of increased milk production. However, this is not painful nor does it prevent the infant from feeding.

Nursing mothers should drink at least two quarts of liquid each day.   Research has shown that drinking extra fluid does not increase milk production but rather decreases milk production. Excessive fluid intake is uncomfortable. Nursing mothers should drink to thirst.

My milk never came in.   The first few days, the baby receives colostrum. Feeding should be frequent because the baby's stomach is small and can only tolerate small amounts at a time. The high number of feedings often leads the mother to think she does not have any milk. In actuality, colostrum is produced as early as the third month of pregnancy. Colostrum continues to be produced through the second week of the infant's life. The amount of colostrum gradually declines as the amount of mature milk increases.

Women with flat or inverted nipples cannot breastfeed.   When inverted nipples are discovered prenatally, the use of Hoffman's exercises or breast shells may help most causes of inverted nipples. If inversion is discovered postpartum, shells can be used between feedings to encourage the nipples to protrude. In most cases, women with inverted nipples can breastfeed using techniques such as the nipple sandwich and electric pump to facilitate latch-on.

Women with small breasts may not make enough milk.   The fatty tissue of the breast determines breast size. Fatty tissue is not involved in milk production or milk flow. Breast size does not influence milk production.

Babies need water, glucose water, and supplemental feedings until the mother's milk "comes in."   There is no evidence that warrants the use of glucose water or supplemental feeding. Colostrum has 17 kcal/oz, glucose water has 6 kcal/oz, and sterile water has 0 kcal. Therefore, colostrum prevents weight loss. Further, supplemental feedings lead to reduced breastfeeds and reduced milk production. Use of supplemental feedings can also lead to nipple confusion and ineffective sucking. Colostrum is a natural substance and is not irritating if aspirated, unlike glucose water that can irritate the lungs. Furthermore, the higher protein levels of colostrum prevent hypoglycemia, having a more stabilizing effect on blood glucose levels than glucose water.

Breastfeeding does not protect against jaundice; if the baby gets jaundice, he or she needs water to reduce the bilirubin concentration.   Jaundice is caused by an accumulation of bilirubin in the infant's system and gives the infant a yellow color to the skin. Neonatal "physiologic" jaundice is considered normal and generally appears around day two or three. Colostrum acts as a laxative, reducing bilirubin recirculation through the gut wall. Water does not have the same laxative action as colostrum and is a less effective treatment for jaundice.

Babies have to work harder when breastfeeding than when sucking from a bottle. Babies do not work harder when breastfeeding if they are positioned correctly. The breast responds to the baby's sucking with milk ejection. Breastfeeding encourages an absence of deviations in patterns of transcutaneous oxygen during breastfeeding, unlike bottle feeding which causes deviation in transcutaneous oxygen patterns.

Infants need extra water during hot weather.   Studies show that breastfed infants manage well without additional water.

Human milk is low in iron; therefore, infants need iron supplements.   A full-term baby is born with at least a four- to six-month store of iron. Free iron may encourage the growth of pathologic bacteria and causes diarrhea and other bowel disorders. Human milk iron is bound to lactoferrin, transferrin, and citrate, releasing only when the infant needs the iron, keeping it from being used by unwanted bacteria. Furthermore, iron in formula is absorbed less efficiently than iron from human milk.

An occasional bottle of formula does not hurt.   Giving an infant a bottle means the infant misses a nursing session, resulting in possible engorgement if the milk is not expressed, which takes more time than breastfeeding. Formula takes longer to digest than human milk, disrupting the baby's built-in feeding "schedule" by postponing the next feeding. In very young infants, use of a bottle can result in possible nipple confusion.

Marketing Breastfeeding

"Markets are not created by God, nature or economic forces, but by businessmen. There may have been no customer want at all until business created it—by advertising, by salesmanship, or by inventing something new. In every case, it is business action that creates the customer" (Drucker, 1974).

DEVELOPING A MARKETING PLAN

An effective marketing plan is essential to successful use of any product or service by the consumer. The marketing plan must describe the benefits and values of breastfeeding. A brief statement telling how breastfeeding has been used in the past, the current uses, and desired future use is necessary to develop a marketing plan. Steps must be identified to implement the marketing plan. The impact of external factors—such as socioeconomic, political, and legal issues—and racial, cultural, and geographic locations influence the success of marketing plans. The appropriate audiences that will promote and use breastfeeding must be identified. The proper use of media techniques and the method to measure media effectiveness must be determined. Most important, an appropriate message identifying the product must be developed, one that is honest and builds trust for the end user. (See Table 1A–9.)

Purpose and Benefits

It is essential that a central theme that describes the purpose and benefits of breastfeeding be developed. The theme should create a visual picture that can be seen in the present and future. Governmental health organizations from every part of the world recognize that breastfeeding is the best source of food and drink for newborn infants during the first six months of life. A logo that is easy to understand, identifies breastfeeding as best, and will attract new users well into the future should be developed. This assists in packaging the idea of breastfeeding and packaging is the primary physical means of influencing human behavior.

Table 1A–9   How Can Health-Care Professionals Encourage Breastfeeding?

1. By acknowledging that breastmilk and formula are not equivalent. By waking up to the reality that by presenting it this way we are harming the future health of not only our nation's youth but the world as a result of our influence.
2. By acknowledging that health outcomes differ depending on whether an infant is breastfed or formula fed.
3. By working to change policies and practices in health-care facilities so that breastfeeding is encouraged and assistance is available.
4. By ensuring contact between mother and infant is uninterrupted during the first hour after birth or until the first breastfeeding has been accomplished.

Source: Walker, M. (1992). Why aren't more mothers breastfeeding? *Childbirth Instr, Winter.* Used with permission.

Past, Present, and Future Use

A situational analysis must be completed to determine the past, present, and future use of breastfeeding. An analysis of the strengths and weaknesses of the market and the competing products' share of the market are necessary to project future use and establish goals. There are many products and baby milk manufacturers in the global market today have used competitive analysis to develop markets to compete with breastfeeding. Therefore, efforts must be made to effectively demonstrate and capitalize on the strengths of breastfeeding, including nutritional benefits, anti-infective, and child-spacing effects. Perceived weaknesses by health-care professionals and consumers must be minimized to increase breastfeeding of newborn infants.

Internal and Exernal Factors to Consider in the Situational Analysis

The internal factors of breastfeeding are the feelings that influence the mother's decision. Some of the internal factors that have been discussed include lack of confidence in ability, lack of education about lactation mechanics, disapproval by significant others, anticipated loss of freedom, and embarrassment. External factors related to breastfeeding are the factors that are beyond the mother's control. The effects of external factors, such as economic conditions, political issues, and regulatory considerations, must be carefully considered. Technology also plays a role in breastfeeding. Economic conditions resulting in a worldwide economic downturn have created a demand for baby milk producers to provide products that meet higher standards than previously required. Because of the various array of baby milk products, competition between the baby milk producers is keen.

The political aspects of breastfeeding are complex and will continue to be a significant external factor in the mother's choice to breastfeed. Pharmaceutical companies and baby milk producers often provide research and grant funds to hospitals. In some cases, these companies donate equipment needed by hospitals to provide the most recent, up-to-date means to treat patients. Health-care providers feel that they should be loyal to these companies and, therefore, often unconsciously, do not place a strong emphasis on breastfeeding.

Regulatory considerations are very important, particularly in the case of working mothers who are not allowed time during the workday to breastfeed their infants. In addition, a proper environment is not provided for mothers to breastfeed infants at work or in many public places.

Technological advances have changed the way today's society lives. The pace of life is much faster, rapidly changing, and places increasing demands on a mother's time-management ability.

Identifying the Appropriate Markets

Following completion of the situational analysis, goals must be established, market segmentation determined, alternative markets reviewed, and selection of target markets identified. Failure to determine the appropriate markets will result in an ineffective marketing plan and lower consumer use.

Segmenting the Market

By segmenting the market, prospective users or supporters possessing a common goal are reached by specific marketing methods. This group of users will respond to the marketing methods based on the common need or goal. One common goal connecting breastfeeding groups is the well-being of the newborn infant. In addition, other segmenting variables, such as regional influences, family size, lifestyles, and benefits offered to the customers, should be taken into account. For example, rural mothers who do not work may be more willing to breastfeed than urban mothers who do not work because urban mothers have more available options to choose from during the day, such as attending social club meetings, libraries, or museums. Mothers of large families may feel they do not have the time to breastfeed a newborn because of the time they spend trying to manage a household.

Analyzing Alternative Opportunities

Analyzing alternative market opportunities allows product strategies to be developed that create expansion of the product's use by increasing market penetration. Extensive market development through introducing the product in new markets can increase usage.

After reviewing the alternative marketing opportunities, one or more target markets must be identified as the basis for development of the marketing program. To increase the breastfeeding market, two obvious groups to target would be first-time mothers and health-care professionals.

STEPS TO IMPLEMENT THE MARKETING PLAN

The target market segments form the basis for the marketing plan. In addition, the goals, budget, and timing must be determined. The marketing plan leads to the implementation process. Implementation involves the two-step process of executing the marketing plan and designing the marketing organization.

Setting Goals

Goals should focus on a group of targeted customers who need, want, and desire the use of a product (breastmilk, breast pumps) or service (breastfeeding assistance). The customers, if from a segment of the market, will respond somewhat similarly to the marketing techniques used. Attention should be given to how the goal will be obtained by focusing the message on the targeted customers' needs, wants, and desires.

Planning and Developing Strategies

The use of good planning techniques and proper research data will enable the selection of good targeted markets. Expected growth, competitive position, the cost of reaching the segment, compatibility with the breastfeeding objective, and resources need to be analyzed to ensure that breastfeeding goals are achieved.

Executing the Plan

Strategies must be developed to achieve the marketing goals. Attention to details is critically important on a daily basis. The day-to-day decisions are referred to as marketing tactics and are crucial to strategic success. Because of continuous global market changes, an effective marketing organization is required to plan, research, sell, and promote the product or service.

Effective Marketing Organization

To effectively operate the marketing program, a marketing organization must be established. There are four main areas: planning, marketing research, sales, and promotion. The marketing organization's goal is to take the marketing plan and make it work. Results of the marketing plan must be compared to the written goals. Discrepancies must be identified and corrective action taken.

Analyzing Market Results

To identify the action required to improve weaknesses or take advantage of marketing strengths, results must be analyzed to compare the goals with the end results. When results show discrepancies, whether positive or negative, action must be taken. In the case of positive results, it is necessary to discover the reason for the better-than-planned-for results and incorporate the results in future planning. Negative results require that revised planning occur to correct appropriate areas.

USING THE MEDIA

Careful consideration must be given to the right advertising media to use and the choices of marketing vehicles within each advertising media. Generally a mix of marketing vehicles is used to maximize the exposure of the product to the targeted market segment. Another consideration is the amount of the advertising budget and projected costs.

Choosing the Right Mix

The types of media selected must be related to the targeted audience, the nature of the message, budget constraints, and campaign objectives. The primary goal of the media mix is to maximize the exposure while minimizing the cost. The reach, rating, and frequency of the message must be analyzed. The different media include television, radio, magazines, newspapers, direct mail, and outdoor advertising.

Selecting the Media Mix

Choosing the media mix is complex and must be looked at based on several factors. It is important to know what the media habits of the targeted market audience are. Low-income groups typically rely on television and word of mouth. Higher-income groups rely on newspapers, personal libraries, public libraries, and television. The product attributes may influence what media are used. Cost is also a factor.

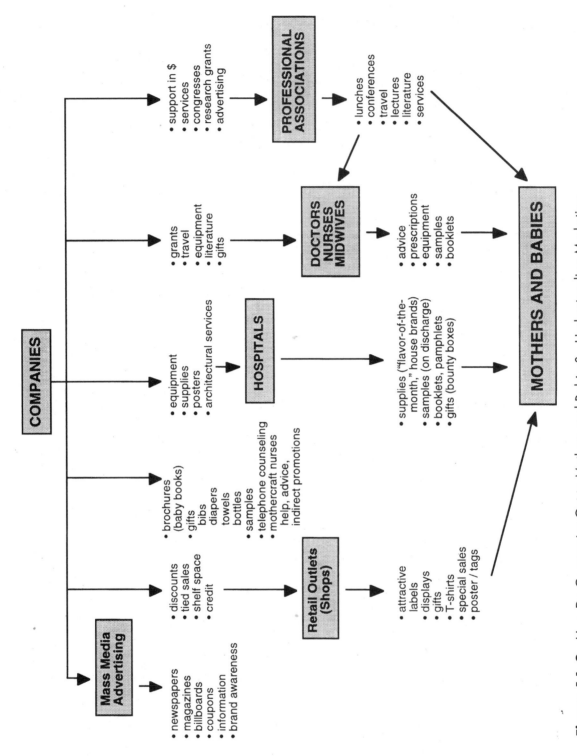

Figure 1A-2 How Do Companies Get to Mothers and Babies?—Understanding Marketing

Source: Adapted from Mantel, J. (1989). International Code of Marketing of Breastmilk Substitutes: What is happening? In Baumslag, N. & Putney, P. (Eds.), *Breastfeeding: A Passport to Life* (p. 59). NGO Committee, UNICEF, New York. Reprinted with permission.

Scheduling the Advertising

There are three approaches to scheduling advertising. These are the steady or regularly scheduled advertisements, the intermittent schedule, and the burst schedule. All three approaches are applicable to marketing breastfeeding.

A steady scheduling needs to be used for health-care providers and professionals to increase awareness by reminding physicians, nurses, and other health professionals regularly that breastfeeding is a viable option for the newborn infant. This will increase the discussion of breastfeeding among expectant mothers. The intermittent schedule will allow additional information to be provided to expectant mothers as there is a need for the information. The burst schedule is the best schedule for marketing breastfeeding because it is a combination of the steady schedule and intermittent schedule that is used primarily during heavy periods of promotion.

Evaluating the Advertising Program

An effective advertising program is evaluated before and after the advertising is used. This is required to ensure that the advertisements are accomplishing their purpose. One way to accomplish evaluation would be to use one survey designed for health-care providers and professionals and another survey for mothers of newborn infants. Another way would be to use inquiry tests that offer additional product information to the advertisement's viewers or readers.

POST-TEST

For questions 1 to 5, choose the best answer.

1. Feeding of supplemental foods to infants
   A. was first proposed by the dairy industry.
   B. has been in place for thousands of years.
   C. is a result of the artificial baby milk market.
   D. does not occur in most developing countries.

2. In the early twentieth century, it was common for manufacturers
   A. to seek uses for the surplus of cow's milk.
   B. to recommend the feeding of prepackaged artificial baby milks.
   C. to employ wet nurses for hire.
   D. to question the practice of breastfeeding as outdated.

3. Breastfeeding rates were lowest in _____, began to rise and hit a plateau in the mid to late _____, and ascended again in the early _____.
   A. early fifties, sixties, seventies
   B. early eighties, eighties, nineties
   C. late forties, fifties, eighties
   D. early seventies, eighties, nineties

4. Behavior and social change are led by the _____, with the _____ the last to make a change.
   A. urban poor, urban elite
   B. urban elite, rural poor

C. rural poor, middle class

D. middle class, urban elite

5. Which of the following is believed to have contributed to the rise of artificial feeding as the norm in the United States?

A. Decrease in geographic mobility

B. Increase in small nuclear families and decrease in multigenerational families

C. Increase in multigenerational families and in breastfeeding role models

D. Shortage of cow's milk

For questions 6 to 10, choose the best answer from the following key:

A. 1990   D. 1992

B. 1982   E. 1989

C. 1994

6. The year the USDA issued the final rule that requires the development of general standards to measure that WIC programs adequately support and promote breastfeeding.

7. The year of the Convention on the Rights of the Child.

8. The year the Breastfeeding Promotion Act was signed in the United States.

9. The year the FDA published formula quality-control regulations in the United States.

10. The year the United States voted for the WHO Code of Marketing of Breast-milk Substitutes.

For questions 11 to 15, choose the best answer.

11. The traditional phase of social and behavioral change is defined

A. as the phase in which prevalence falls and duration becomes shorter.

B. as the phase in which high prevalence and duration of a change occurs after early promotional efforts.

C . as the phase of rising prevalence and duration which follows the transformation phase.

D. as the phase of decreasing duration but rising prevalence.

12. The _____ the maternal age, the _____ the incidence of breastfeeding in the United States.

A. higher, lower

B. lower, higher

C. lower, lower

D. higher, higher

13. A cultural idea about breastfeeding, which proposes that women nurse babies other than their own to promote alliances and peace with enemy tribes, strengthen unity, and create family bonds to prevent marriage, is called

A. baraka.

B. milk sharing.

C. milk kinship.

D. trust transfer.

14. The incidence of breastfeeding is likely to be highest in which of these groups?

    A. New immigrants

    B. Adolescents

    C. WIC participants

    D. Women with income >$25,000

15. Increases in incidence from 1989 to 1993 have been reported for which group?

    A. New immigrants

    B. Unmarried, high-income women

    C. Employed women

    D. WIC participants

For questions 16 to 20, choose the best answer from the following:

    A. if responses 1, 2, and 3 are correct   **D. if response 4 is correct**

    B. if responses 1 and 3 are correct   **E. if all are correct**

    C. if responses 2 and 4 are correct

16. Barriers to breastfeeding include

    1. lack of support, too many rules.

    2. too many rules, embarrassment.

    3. embarrassment, loss of freedom.

    4. supportive families, flexible work schedules.

17. External factors that influence a marketing plan include

    1. feelings that influence the mother's decision.

    2. political and legal issues in the marketplace.

    3. conscious ambivalence toward breastfeeding by health-care workers.

    4. economic conditions in the marketplace.

18. Determining the appropriate market for a product or service will result in

    1. lack of markets for the product or service.

    2. an effective marketing plan.

    3. unsuccessful results for the growth of the product or service.

    4. higher consumer use of the product or service.

19. To maximize the exposure of the product or service to the targeted market

    1. a mix of marketing vehicles is used.

    2. the mix of media should be carefully chosen.

    3. the media habits of the targeted market audience must be known.

    4. an evaluation of the advertising program should be conducted.

20. Media mix selection should take _____ into consideration.

    1. the media habits of the targeted audience

    2. the product attributes

    3. the cost of the media

    4. global market changes

SECTION B

The Impact of Breastfeeding on the Family and Community

Jill L. Goode, RD/LD
Donna Calhoun, BS, IBCLC

LEARNING OBJECTIVES

At the completion of this section, the learner will be able to do the following:

1. Discuss the changes in family relationships that occur with the birth of a child.
2. Discuss the impact of breastfeeding on the father and describe his role in caring for the mother–infant dyad.
3. Discuss extended family members' roles and concerns when breastfeeding is the infant-feeding choice.
4. Discuss the difficulties that returning to work after the birth of a baby can present for the breastfeeding family.
5. Describe practical suggestions to ease the transition to work for the breastfeeding family.

OUTLINE

   I. Changes in Interfamilial Relationships

      A. Baby-centered focus

      B. Attachment Parenting

         1. Infant attachment checklist

         2. Parental behaviors

II. Father's Role in the Breastfeeding Relationship

   A. Preparing fathers for breastfeeding

   B. Meeting fathers' needs

III. Extended Family Members' Roles

IV. Postpartum and Self-Esteem Issues

V. When Women Work Outside the Home

   A. Why breastfeed when returning to employment?

   B. Obstacles to breastfeeding in the workplace

   C. Tips for successfully combining work and breastfeeding

PRE-TEST

For questions 1 to 4, choose the best answer.

1. Unrestricted breastfeeding
   A. occurs when infants are put to breast on cue with no offering of bottles of artificial supplementation.
   B. is when guidelines dictate the frequency and duration of feeds.
   C. results in additional feeds of artificial milk.
   D. is practiced in most industrialized countries today.

2. Responsiveness to the individual child via attachment parenting is evidenced by which of the following practices?
   A. Maintaining separate sleep arrangements for the baby
   B. Practicing token breastfeeding
   C. Responding to your baby's cues
   D. Increasing time spent together as a couple

3. All of the following will enhance the transition to parenting for the father except:
   A. providing anticipatory guidance about breastfeeding.
   B. supporting the couple's adult relationship.
   C. having the father assume basic infant care.
   D. enhancing the father–infant relationship.

4. Changes in interfamilial relationships that occur after delivery in families practicing unrestricted breastfeeding include a shift
   A. to token breastfeeding.
   B. away from attachment parenting.
   C. to sibling-centered family focus.
   D. to a baby-centered family focus.

For questions 5 to 8, choose the best answer from the following key:

    A. Low-risk infant attachment   **B. High-risk infant attachment**

5. Infant can fixate on mother's eyes and develops good following response.

6. Weak contact in eye-following response.

7. Weak crying response or rageful, tearless crying.

8. Infant will respond to mother's positive nurturing.

For questions 9 to 12, choose the best answer from the following key:

    A. Low-risk parenting   **B. High-risk parenting**

9. Mother provides infant with proper and preventive medical assistance.

10. Baby is overstimulated by too much talking and touching by the mother.

11. Mother wants to hold, caress, and respond to infant's vocalization.

12. Mother shows minimal touching, stroking, or talking to or about baby.

For questions 13 to 15, choose the best answer.

13. Obstacles to breastfeeding in the workplace include
    A. extended maternity leave.
    B. onsite child care.
    C. uniform labor standards that protect all women.
    D. lack of facilities and time to express breastmilk.

14. The largest increase in the labor force is in
    A. women over age 45.
    B. men with children under 5 years of age.
    C. women with infants and toddlers.
    D. men between 15 and 44 years of age.

15. Mother-friendly workplaces may provide
    A. shortened maternity leaves.
    B. on-premises day care.
    C. fewer breaks.
    D. inflexible schedules.

For questions 16 to 20, choose the best answer from the following key:

    A. Supportive of combining breastfeeding and working
    B. Not supportive of combining breastfeeding and working

16. Discuss your infant feeding decision with your supervisor, outlining several options of how to implement your plan.

17. Begin pumping your first day back to work.

18. Discuss your feeding plans with the infant's caregiver so the infant can be fed immediately prior to your return to pick him or her up.

19. Returning to work on a Thursday or Friday to ease the separation period.

20. Delaying the return to work as long as possible.

Changes in Interfamilial Relationships

Breastfeeding is an integral part of the reproductive process, the natural and ideal way of feeding the infant, and a unique biological and emotional basis for child development. In the breastfeeding process, the family is provided with a method to ease the stress that naturally accompanies the addition of a new baby to the family equation. The infant's primary needs are met when he or she is brought to the mother's breast. Breastfeeding allows for a smooth transition from uterine to extrauterine life. Mothers who breastfeed can respond to their babies more intuitively and with less hesitation, and without delay (Sears & Sears, 1993).

BABY-CENTERED FOCUS

The classic work of Newton and Newton (1967) regarding the psychosocial nature of breastfeeding gives us a measure of insight into the possible impact of breastfeeding on the family unit. By gaining some knowledge of the breastfeeding mother as different from other mothers (her peers), we can begin to understand how her relationship with her nursing infant affects her relationship with those in her immediate family constellation. The Newtons describe two distinct breastfeeding groups. Unrestricted breastfeeding occurs when the infant is put to the breast on cue, usually greater than 10 times in a 24-hour period. These infants are not offered bottles of artificial supplements, water, or solids until the second half of the first year of life. Breastfeeding remains a major source of nourishment into the second year of life. This group continues to represent a minority in most industrialized countries. On the other hand, token breastfeeding allows guidelines (other than infants' cues) to dictate frequency and duration of feeds. Additional feeds of artificial milk and solids are not unusual. The infant's sucking at the breast is restricted; therefore, the milk ejection reflex is never completely established. Weaning has usually taken place by the third month.

In a family where unrestricted breastfeeding is practiced, the interfamilial relationships shift as the new baby's needs become the focal point. This shift forces change in the existing relationships. Siblings must share their parents and less time may be available to meet their needs. Siblings will reflect their mother's attitude about breastfeeding and parenting.

ATTACHMENT PARENTING

The following are five tools to use:

1. Connect with your baby early.
2. Read and respond to your baby's cues.
3. Breastfeed your baby.
4. Wear your baby (use a sling to carry your baby).
5. Share sleep arrangements with your baby.

If the mother is relaxed and secure about her role, the older children will reflect this ease (Lawrence, 1989). William and Martha Sears (1993) suggest a "high touch" form of parenting that entails being responsive to the individual child; this is called attachment parenting. Breastfeeding is listed as one of the tools of this style of parenting. Attachment parenting can, eventually, make the parents' job easier and may have lifelong effects on the entire family unit (Sears & Sears, 1993). The model of attachment parenting is assimilated by the older children in the family, easing the acceptance of the newborn into the family unit (Sears & Sears, 1993). Infant attachment is discussed in more detail in Module 4, *The Management of Breastfeeding*, Chapter 1.

Infant Attachment Checklist*

Low-Risk Signs
- Infant cries to signal unmet need and when gratified will gradually terminate crying.
- Infant may resist cuddling sometimes but with moderate touching and body sculpturing, infant will positively respond to mother's positive nurturing.
- Baby can fixate on mother's eyes and develops good following response, especially when nursing or smiling.
- Infant may have some nursing difficulty (mother's nursing difficulty because of inverted nipples, etc.) but can adapt and quickly develop healthy responses.
- Baby gurgles, chortles, and has smiling response, especially when primary caregiver smiles.

High-Risk Signs
- Weak crying response or rageful crying (without tears) and/or constantly whining.
- Poor clinging and extreme resistance to cuddling and close holding (fights to get free). Arches back when picked up (after first six weeks of life) and seems "stiff as a board."
- Weak contact in eye-following response. Infant will highly resist close face-to-face eye contact and consistently avert gaze (even if cuddling is permitted).
- Baby has poor suckling response and isn't motivated to approach mother for nurturing. Can also be caused by developmental difficulties (e.g., cleft palate).
- Infants resist smiles even when tickled or played with lovingly. No reciprocal smile response.

Parental Behaviors*

Low-Risk Parenting
- Mother exhibits positive interest in baby at birth and is eager to interact.
- Mother wants to hold, caress, and respond to infant's vocalization. Makes positive statements about baby, "She's adorable."

*Adapted from Magid, K and C. McKelvey (1987). *High Risk: Children Without a Conscience*, p. 248. New York: Bantam Books. Used with permission.

- Happy mother is filled with radiance, even, at times, tears of joy.
- Mother is attuned with baby's need for a balance of stimulation and quiet time. They develop a healthy rhythm of play and rest together.
- Mother frequently establishes face-to-face positioning with eye contact and appropriate smiles.
- Mother plays with infant when awake (but doesn't overdo it) and places baby in stimulating area to observe and interact with others. Shows ability to comfort child and appears strongly attached.
- Mother provides infant with proper and preventive medical assistance. Concern for diet, diaper changes, and health of baby.
- Mother is basically happy and satisfied with being a mother and primary caregiver.

High-Risk Parenting
- Mother withdraws and assumes a negative psychological and physical posture regarding baby at birth.
- Minimal touching, stroking, or talking to or about baby unless in negative manner. "Be quiet." May hold infant tensely.
- Emotionless and flat affect or depressed and angry. Sometimes tears of sadness.
- Mother overstimulates baby by too much talking and touching. Mother sometimes plays in inappropriate or hostile ways (cruelly teasing infant).
- Mother doesn't establish eye contact except when angry and rarely smiles or does so inappropriately (when infant is in pain).
- Leaves infant, when awake, for long periods in isolation and doesn't show the ability to comfort the baby when needed. Handles baby roughly or in detached manner and may be abusive and neglectful.
- Mother fails to provide basic supplies for well-baby care and is angry at most baby behaviors. Mother doesn't seek medical assistance unless a crisis occurs.
- Mother is unhappy, frustrated, and angry at being a mother and the primary caregiver.

Father's Role in the Breastfeeding Relationship

Father finds himself in the position of nurturing the mother while striving to establish his own bond with the new infant. Often the father's role in the breastfeeding family is overlooked by those caring for the mother and baby. By giving attention to the ways in which the close mother–baby bond of the breastfeeding relationship influences the father, caregivers can enhance the parenthood transition and help to foster strong father–infant bonds.

PREPARING FATHERS FOR BREASTFEEDING

Jordan and Wall (1993) have identified several areas of intervention for fathers concerning breastfeeding. They are:

1. **Provide anticipatory guidance about breastfeeding:**
   - Include the father in prenatal education to bridge the gap between expectations and reality.
   - Provide an opportunity for fathers to express fears and to ask questions in an all-male environment with trained and experienced fathers of breastfed children.

2. **Support the couple's adult relationship:**
   - Acknowledge the fundamental value to the family of a strong relationship between the mother and father.
   - Acknowledge some fathers' feelings of displacement by the infant.
   - Suggest ways the couple can maintain communication and intimacy while not compromising the newborn's needs.

3. **Enhance the father–infant relationship:**
   - Give father "permission" to establish his unique close bond with his infant.
   - Promote time for father to master basic infant-care skills and learn his infant's cues.

4. **When couples do not breastfeed exclusively, provide guidelines for increasing fathers' interaction opportunities:**
   - Suggest minimal time of exclusive breastfeeding for mother and baby to master the fundamentals of breastfeeding.
   - Inform parents that initial fussiness and resistance are part of the expected adjustment period.

MEETING FATHERS' NEEDS

It is not at all unusual for fathers to feel left out (Jordan & Wall, 1993), jealous, or resentful of the tremendous amount of emotional and physical energy the new mother has to expend in caring for her newborn. If this is a couple's first baby, the father may not know how to handle his feelings of displacement (Sears & Sears, 1993).

The "couple" that existed before the birth of the baby must experience a metamorphosis. The methods of communication and intimacy often must be adjusted to accommodate the needs of the newborn infant. Mother's sexual intimacy will be affected by breastfeeding, and the intense needs of the newborn often takes new parents by surprise. Mothers are especially prone to feeling "touched out" (Lawrence, 1989; Riordan & Auerbach, 1993) and, therefore, are not as receptive to sexual intimacy with partners. A father who takes advantage of attachment-style fathering is more likely to be sensitive to the new mother's feelings and feel that he is a contributing partner in the new family. This giving of self is emotionally fulfilling and contributes to the forming of the new family.

Extended Family Members' Roles

Breastfeeding is a learned behavior. It can be easily learned though informal teaching in cultures where the majority of women openly breastfeed. However, in the United States, there is a generation of women who have no personal breastfeeding experience. Also, in many cases, where there is a role model for breastfeeding, the family structure is such that access to this person is unlikely. We now have small nuclear families with fewer generations living in the same house. This change in the family structure has resulted in the lack of available and/or knowledgeable female relatives who are able to provide breastfeeding guidance. Consumers now look to health-care providers for breastfeeding information and guidance.

Family members and close friends influence the decision to combine breastfeeding and work by viewing breastfeeding as a home activity, embarrassing, and/or incompatible with employment (Auerbach & Guss, 1984). Targeting the significant family member with educational interventions to teach how to support the breastfeeding dyad may help strengthen chances for a positive and rewarding breastfeeding experience for mother and infant.

Postpartum and Self-Esteem Issues

Physical and emotional changes occur in the mother that, hopefully, can be handled through preventive care and anticipatory guidance. Not all women are able to have early prenatal care with close monitoring. Issues such as contraception, diet, and maternal medications can influence breastfeeding. Detailed discussions of these issues can be found in Module 3, *The Science of Breastfeeding*, Chapter 2, and Module 4, *The Management of Breastfeeding*, Chapter 2.

A successful birth experience encourages the successful development of the maternal role. Laufer (1990) suggests that women who have very negative birth experiences feel a loss in self-esteem that can be recovered via successful breastfeeding. Self-esteem is a product of a lifetime of experiences. Components of self-esteem—significance, competence, connectedness—are balanced by separation, realism, ethics, and values in an interactive process. Challenges to self-esteem that women face include the following:

- A lack of sufficient self-knowledge
- Self-concept dislocation
- Self-concept constricted by cultural understanding of role and gender
- Completely negative self-concept
- Lack of structural balance in self-concept
- Ideal image in transition

When appropriate, the lactation consultant can try some or all of the following to raise maternal self-esteem: touch, praise, encouragement, illusion bashing, acceptance, "I" messages versus judgment, structure, listening, providing realistic pictures of maternal role, targeting social support systems.

When Women Work Outside the Home

Labor force increases in the United States are highest for women in the childbearing years who have infants and toddlers (Bureau of National Affairs Special Report, 1986). The 1990 population records indicate 56,554,000 women were in the civilian labor force and 72% of them were in the childbearing ages of 16 to 44 years (Bureau of Census, 1992). The women most likely to choose breastfeeding are also more likely to return to paid employment outside the home (Martinez et al., 1981; Ryan & Martinez, 1989). Continuing to breastfeed after returning to work or school can be a challenge, but with some good advice and support, women can successfully combine breastfeeding and an active lifestyle.

WHY BREASTFEED WHEN RETURNING TO EMPLOYMENT?

Breastfed infants are much healthier than formula-fed infants both physically and emotionally. Breastmilk provides all of an infant's nutritional needs for the first six months of life. The baby's immune system is strengthened by the ingredients in breastmilk. Breastfed infants have fewer respiratory-tract infections, ear infections, and diarrhea than formula-fed infants; breastfed infants also have fewer food allergies. Because breastfeeding supports bonding and development of long-lasting feelings of love and security, breastfed babies may be emotionally healthier. The benefits are more clearly outlined in Chapter 2 of this module.

There are many benefits for the working mother who breastfeeds. The bond between mother and infant is strengthened by breastfeeding. This is especially important to women who are separated from their infants by work. Breastfeeding helps the uterus return to its prepregnancy state more quickly. Women who breastfeed are less likely to develop ovarian and breast cancers and osteoporosis. Breastfeeding helps women develop a sense of confidence and self-reliance. Women who breastfeed experience both physical and emotional benefits.

Breastfeeding also benefits the family as a whole. Breastfeeding costs less than formula feeding, taking less out of the budget and allowing more resource availability to the rest of the family. Also, breastfeeding requires less preparation time and is more convenient; so, there is more of mother's time for other family members.

A 1989 profile of breastfeeding and the working mother reveals that only 10% of mothers who are employed full-time and are breastfeeding at hospital discharge will continue through six months, whereas 24% of breastfeeding mothers not employed will reach six months. Of the total births in 1992 for one utility company with a corporate lactation program in place, 29% (29/100) of the women delivering returned to work breastfeeding and pumping and 23% (23/100) continued through six months (Cohen & Mrtek, 1994). Looking at two corporate lactation programs, 71.3% (77/108) and 78.5% (62/79) of the women who returned to work breastfeeding continued until the child was at least six months old (Cohen & Mrtek, 1994).

Employers who encourage and support breastfeeding find it beneficial. Women who breastfeed tend to be more health-conscious and healthier, decreasing absenteeism as a result of illness. Breastfed infants are healthier, costing the company less in health care and maternal sick leave (see Table 1B–1). Ninety-three percent of infants of mothers at the Los Angeles Department of Water and Power fed formula were ill during a 2-year study compared to 59% of their breastfed counterparts (*News Wave*, 1993). Also, employee morale and productivity may increase in companies who encourage women to breastfeed (Cohen & Mrtek, 1994).

The environment and economy benefit from breastfeeding. Less waste is created by breastfeeding, and what is created is generally biodegradable. Health sectors save money by not buying formula and bottles.

Table 1B–1   Conditions for Which Breastfeeding May Have a Protective Effect: Impact on Work Days Lost and Treatment Costs

Conditions	Range of Cost for Treatment[1]	No. Days off for Employee[2]	Effects of Breastfeeding	References
Diarrhea	$50–$70 (mild) $1500–$3000 (severe)	1–5	3- to 4-fold decrease in risk; less likely to be hospitalized	Duffy et al., 1986; Howie et al., 1990; Palti et al., 1984; Fallot et al., 1980
Ear Infections	$60–$80	1–2	Up to 60% decrease in risk	Duncan et al., 1993; Chandra, 1979; Teele et al., 1989; Saarinen, 1982
Ear Tubes	$400–$1650	2–3		
Bronchitis/Pneumonia (lower respiratory infection)	$60–$80 (mild) $4600–$5000 (severe)	2–7	Up to 80% decrease in risk; less likely to be hospitalized	Leventhal et al., 1986; Wright et al., 1989; Fallot et al., 1980
Allergies (food)	$400 (diagnosis) $80–$100 (acute reaction treatment)	1–2 (per reaction)	4- to 5-fold decrease in allergic symptoms	Chandra, 1979; Merrett et al., 1988; Harris et al., 1989; Chandra, 1992
Respiratory Syncytial Virus (upper and lower)	$60–$80 (mild) $4600–$5000 (hospitalized)	2–7	Less likely to be hospitalized	Pullan et al., 1980
Meningitis	$4500–$32,000	3 days to 3 weeks	4-fold decrease in risk; decrease in severity	Cochi et al., 1986; Takala et al., 1989; Fallot et al., 1980
Baby Bottle Tooth Decay	$250 (cleaning/repair) $3000 (replacement)	1–4	Very low risk	Abbey, 1979
Insulin-Dependent Diabetes Mellitus	$3000–$5000 (without complications)	5–15	Reduced risk of trigger through cow's milk proteins	Karjalainen et al., 1992; Mayer et al., 1988; Virtanen et al., 1991

[1]Average cost for treatment in Lexington, KY, in 1993. Includes cost of regular office visit(s), medication, and normal hospitalization.

[2]Average number of days a child would be too ill to go to child-care center per illness episode, resulting in loss of work days for a parent.

Source: Developed in 1993 by Doraine Bailey, MA, Lexington-Fayette County Health Department, 650 Newtown Pike, Lexington, KY 40508. Reprinted with permission.

OBSTACLES TO BREASTFEEDING IN THE WORKPLACE

Some women face serious obstacles when trying to return to work while breast-feeding. The obstacles to breastfeeding, as identified by the World Alliance for Breastfeeding Action (WABA) in *Mother-Friendly Workplace Initiative Action Folder* (1993), include:

1. Maternity leave may only be available to certain employees.
2. Women who work in agriculture, domestic jobs, and other informal work sectors are not covered by government-enforced standards.
3. Employers may preferentially hire males if they must foot the entire bill for leave and child care.
4. Child-care facilities and breaks to breastfeed are not available for many workers in small companies or in nonformal work settings.
5. Maternal benefits are viewed as extras rather than an entitlement or investment in health.
6. National socioeconomic conditions (poverty, debt, etc.) consume resources leaving little to support breastfeeding.
7. Women hold low status in many countries and are considered a low priority.
8. Marketing by baby formula and food companies presents their products as the only solution for working women.
9. Work schedules are often inflexible and women find it hard to find time to pump.
10. Many worksites do not have a private place to pump and women end up hiding in supply closets and vacant offices or straddling a toilet while pumping.

TIPS FOR SUCCESSFULLY COMBINING WORK AND BREASTFEEDING

Preparation is the key to successfully returning to work and continuing to breast-feed:

1. Begin preparing before the infant's birth. Know the legal provisions for maternity leave and the policies your company has. After gathering all the information, prioritize and formulate several plans, from best- to worse-case scenarios. Present your plan, best-case scenario, to your employer before the infant is born (Dana & Price, 1987). Explain the benefits of breastfeeding to your employer. Explore the possible options such as extended maternity leave, part-time work for a period, job sharing, flexible hours, or working at home for your employer.
2. Select a caregiver. Explore the many child-care options, such as a babysitter in the home, day care, nanny, relatives caring for infants and weigh the pros and cons before selecting one that meets your needs (Dana & Price, 1987). Ensure that the person who is to care for the infant understands and supports breastfeeding (WABA, 1993). Give the caregiver explicit written instructions on how to store breastmilk (WABA, 1993).

3. Take as much maternity leave as possible to ensure breastfeeding is well established before returning to work (WABA, 1993). Practice pumping at least several weeks before returning to work (Imperiale, 1993). Build up a freezer "breastmilk bank" from the breastmilk collected during practice (Grams, 1985).

4. Find the right pump. All pumps work similarly, creating a vacuum to draw milk out of the breast and collect it in a collection vessel. There are basically three types of pumps: manual, battery-operated, and electric. Consider the cost, portability, and efficiency when selecting a pump. Some women find it difficult to use store-bought, battery-operated pumps and find larger "hospital-grade" electrical pumps easier to use. Also, consider how easy it will be to clean the pump. Using a double-pumping kit may help increase the efficiency and decrease pumping time.

5. Arrange feeding times that work with your schedule. Ask the caregiver not to feed the infant within a couple of hours before your return. Breastfeed more at night when you are away from the infant for long hours during the day.

6. Arrange for help (hired, family, and/or friends) with the housework. Also, prioritize what is important and what is not (Dana & Price, 1987).

7. Find a support group. Local hospital maternity units or international breastfeeding support groups are very helpful (Imperiale, 1993).

8. Introduce the bottle to the baby (Dana & Price, 1987) prior to your return to work.

9. Return to work on a Thursday or Friday, if possible, easing into the separation period (Grams, 1985).

For other useful information, refer to Table 1B–2.

Table 1B–2   Research-based Recommendations to Offer the Employed Breastfeeding Mother

Research Findings	Recommendations
(1) Were most anxious about the baby and breastfeeding the first week of employment	(1) Try to return to work on a Thursday or Friday to be able to look forward to a weekend that is only a day or two away
(2) Waited until the baby was four months or older before returning to work	(2) Stay home as long as possible
(3) Used part-time/flex-time when they first returned	(3) Return on less than a full-time schedule in the beginning
(4) Expressed milk during their absences: (a) especially in the first month (b) to remain physically comfortable (c) to reduce the likelihood of leaking (d) to collect milk for later use	(4) Learn how to express milk
(5) Complained most often about exhaustion	(5) Use breastfeeding as a "break" from home chores
(6) Viewed breastfeeding as the key to continued "connection" with the baby in spite of separations	(6) Remember that only the mother can enjoy the special closeness that breastfeeding represents

Source: Adapted by permission of Elsevier Science Inc. from Assisting the employed breastfeeding mother by K Auerbach, *Journal of Nurse Midwifery*, Vol. 35, No. 1, p. 28. Copyright 1990 by the American College of Nurse-Midwives.

Workplaces are starting to work with women who want to breastfeed. They arrange flexible work schedules and areas for women to breastfeed. Several companies are hiring Corporate Lactation Programs to come in and educate and assist employees who wish to breastfeed and to set up lactation stations (Imperiale, 1993).

WABA (1993) promotes breastfeeding in the context of a mother-friendly workplace. Workplaces that are mother-friendly provide adequate maternity leaves, on-premises day care, alternative work schedules, as well as space and time for practices that support breastfeeding.

POST-TEST

For questions 1 to 4, choose the best answer.

1. Token breastfeeding
   A. describes a method of feeding where no additional feeds of artificial milk are offered.
   B. occurs when guidelines dictate the frequency and duration of feeds and additional feeds of artificial milk are offered.
   C. occurs when infants are fed.
   D. is practiced in most developing countries today.

2. Attachment parenting is a style of parenting that
   A. shifts the focal point of interfamilial relationships to the parents.
   B. encourages a parenting form that is responsive to the individual child.
   C. discourages acceptance of the newborn to the family unit.
   D. threatens older siblings' relationships with their parents.

3. Interventions, which are successful in preparing fathers for breastfeeding, include
   A. discouraging some fathers' feelings of displacement by the infant.
   B. suggesting that a decrease in intimacy and communication between the couple is to be expected for the first few months.
   C. promoting time for father to master basic infant-care skills and learn his infant's cues.
   D. leaving the practice of attachment parenting to the mother.

4. Baby-centered family focus implies
   A. a shift from unrestricted to token breastfeeding.
   B. a style of parenting that emphasizes weaning.
   C. an attachment-parenting style of infant care.
   D. a high-risk parenting style that leads to spoiling.

For questions 5 to 8, choose the best answer from the following key:
   A. Low-risk parenting
   B. High-risk parenting

5. Mother wants to hold, caress, and respond to infant's vocalization.

6. Mother shows minimal touching, stroking, or talking to or about baby.

7. Mother provides infant with proper and preventive medical assistance.

8. Baby is overstimulated by too much talking and touching by the mother.

For questions 9 to 12, choose the best answer from the following key:
   A. Low-risk infant attachment
   B. High-risk infant attachment

9. Infant will respond to mother's positive nurturing.

10. Infant can fixate on mother's eyes and develops good following response.

11. Weak crying response or rageful, tearless crying.

12. Weak contact in eye-following response.

For questions 13 to 15, choose the best answer.

13. Workplaces that facilitate breastfeeding offer
   A. extended maternity leave.
   B. no provision for child care.
   C. no facilities or time to express breastmilk.
   D. labor standards that discriminate against women.

14. Women in the childbearing years of 15 to 44 are
   A. leaving the workforce in record numbers to stay home in the 1990s.
   B. represent the largest growing group entering the workforce in the 1990s.
   C. are second to men aged 15 to 44, as the largest growing group entering the workforce in the 1990s.
   D. are second to men over 55 years in leaving the workforce in the 1990s.

15. Shortened maternity leaves, inflexible schedules, and structured, limited breaks describe workplaces that
   A. are mother friendly.
   B. are baby friendly.
   C. are not mother friendly.
   D. are not baby friendly.

For questions 16 to 20, choose the best answer from the following key:
   A. Supportive of combining breastfeeding and working
   B. Not supportive of combining breastfeeding and working

16. A caregiver who holds off feeding the infant in the immediate period before the mother's return for the infant.

17. Breast-pumping stations at work that are equipped with refrigeration and plumbing.

18. Scheduled, inflexible breaks.

19. Job sharing and extended maternity leaves.

20. Returning to work on the first day of your work week for a full week's schedule of hours.

SECTION C

Prolonging Lactation

Rebecca F. Black, MS, RD/LD, IBCLC
Jill L. Goode, RD/LD
Teresa McCullen, BS, IBCLC

LEARNING OBJECTIVES

At the completion of this section, the learner will be able to do the following:

1. Discuss why prolonging the duration of breastfeeding is important.
2. Discuss the factors influencing breastfeeding duration.
3. Describe community and governmental support programs available for breastfeeding families.
4. Discuss the role of the lactation consultant and other health-care professionals in supporting breastfeeding.
5. Discuss the legal rights of breastfeeding families.

OUTLINE

I. Factors that Influence Lactation Duration

   A. Why extended duration of breastfeeding is important

   B. Breastfeeding definitions

   C. Details on factors influencing duration

II. Community and Social Support

   A. Best Start, Inc.

   B. Public health—Special Supplemental Nutrition Program for Women, Infants, and Children

   C. La Leche League International

D. Peer-counselor programs

E. Breastfeeding educators

F. Lactation consultants

G. Well Start International

III. Legal Issues Surrounding Breastfeeding

PRE-TEST

For questions 1 to 4, choose the best answer.

1. Reasons why dose–response data on breastfeeding has been difficult to collect include all except:

    A. Sophisticated laboratory techniques were not available to detect some breastmilk constituents until the 1970s.

    B. Breastfeeding intensity and frequency by individual women has been consistent over the ages.

    C. Breastfeeding-intensity classification schemes have only recently been described in the literature.

    D. The rapid reduction in duration and intensity that occurred in the late twentieth century make dose–response data difficult to evaluate.

2. One of the first states to pass a law to protect breastfeeding mothers from arrest or harassment as a result of breastfeeding in public.

    A. Georgia

    B. California

    C. Florida

    D. Illinois

3. Breastfeeding in a manner that no other liquid or solid is given to the infant is best described as

    A. high partial breastfeeding.

    B. almost exclusive breastfeeding.

    C. exclusive breastfeeding.

    D. token breastfeeding.

4. Risk factors for shortened duration of breastfeeding include:

    A. Not working, non-WIC participant, not living in the western United States.

    B. Working, WIC participation, not living in the western United States.

    C. Working, non-WIC participant, living in the western United States.

    D. Working, WIC participation, living in the western United States.

For questions 5 to 10, choose the best answer from the following key:

   A. Positively influences duration of breastfeeding

   B. Negatively influences duration of breastfeeding

5. Perceptions of insufficient milk supply

6. Low socioeconomic status, living in the United States

7. Previous breastfeeding experience

8. Rigid feeding schedules

9. Infant/mother sleep separation

10. Residence in a rural community in less developed countries

For questions 11 to 16, choose the best answer from the following key:
   A. La Leche League International
   B. Special Supplemental Nutrition Program for Women, Infants and Children
   C. Best Start
   D. International Lactation Consultant Association
   E. International Board of Lactation Consultant Examiners

11. Provides low-income women and their children with nutrition education and vouchers for food.

12. Develops audiovisual and print materials based on a social marketing concept.

13. Relies on "mother-to-mother" support.

14. World's largest resource on breastfeeding information and support.

15. Is the credentialing agency for lactation consultants.

16. Has published federal regulations on the requirements for breastfeeding promotion and support activities.

For questions 17 to 20, choose the best answer from the following key:
   A. Lactation consultants
   B. Breastfeeding educators
   C. Peer counselors

17. Assists in uncomplicated breastfeeding activities.

18. Breastfeeding mothers helping other breastfeeding mothers.

19. Clinical specialists who can help with complex breastfeeding problems.

20. Concept on which La Leche League International is based.

Factors That Influence Lactation Duration

Prolonging lactation is a goal established by representatives of professional organizations, state public health departments, and private organizations that joined forces at the initial Surgeon General's Workshop on Breastfeeding and Human Lactation in 1984 (U.S. Department of Health and Human Services, Public Health Service). Leading up to and since the establishment of this goal, the factors that influence the duration of lactation have and continue to be researched. Further research is exploring the community and social support of breastfeeding and its influence on duration. Breastfeeding outreach program development is continually taking place. The lactation consultant's role is being defined. The legal rights of breastfeeding mothers are being established via courtroom battles.

Further, the Innocenti Declaration signed in 1990 at the World Summit for Children held in Italy called for all countries to have an appointed breastfeeding coordinator, abide by the WHO code (1981; 1994) which outlines standards of conduct for marketing artificial baby milks, enact legislation protecting the rights of working women, and ensure that every maternity facility fully practices the "Ten Steps to Successful Breastfeeding" (UNICEF, 1992) by 1995. The latter is the foundation for the Baby Friendly Hospital Initiative (BFHI) (UNICEF, 1992).

WHY EXTENDED DURATION OF BREASTFEEDING IS IMPORTANT

Specific studies have reported increasing health benefits of breastfeeding with increased doses. These benefits have been shown for intelligence, malocclusion, gastrointestinal disease and hospitalizations, sudden infant death syndrome (SIDS), and otitis media. See Module 3, *The Science of Breastfeeding*, Chapter 2, for more information.

Reasons why the dose–response data have been so difficult to collect include the following (Fredrickson, Lecture, 1994):

- The analysis of milk constituents requires sophisticated laboratory techniques not available until the 1970s.
- At the turn of the century, breastfeeding was more uniform in duration in the United States and could be a categorical variable. But a rapid reduction in duration and intensity occurred during the later twentieth century, making analysis of dose–response data by epidemiologist/researchers difficult.
- Breastfeeding duration study methodology has only been adopted in the last decade and the intensity classification schemes described in 1990 by Labbok and Krasovec are little used as yet in studies (see Figure 1C-1). In studying breastfeeding, a two-dimensional, continuous variable should be used so that these two questions can be answered:
  1. How many "doses" each day does the infant get of breastmilk?
  2. For how long does the infant get this number of doses?

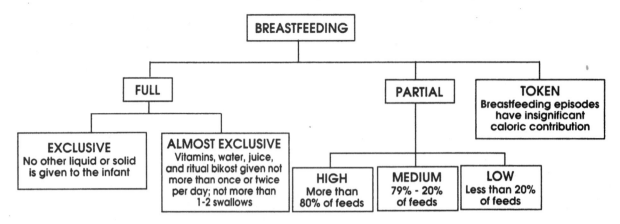

Figure 1C-1   Schema for breastfeeding definition

Source: From Lawrence, R. (1994), *Breastfeeding—A Guide for the Medical Profession*, p. 17. St. Louis: Mosby. Modified from Labbok, M, Krasovec, K (1990). Toward consistency in breastfeeding definitions, *Stud Fam Plann*, 21:226. Reprinted with permission.

BREASTFEEDING DEFINITIONS

The accepted definition of breastfeeding in the past has differentiated token breastfeeding from unrestricted breastfeeding (Newton, 1971). The end result of these two styles is a difference in the duration of breastfeeding, with unrestricted breastfeeding resulting in a longer duration. The Interagency Group for Action on Breastfeeding met in 1988 and standardized terminology for defining breastfeeding behavior. After review, the schema was published (Labbok & Krasovec, 1990).

At the present time, one feeding at the breast is considered the definition of breastfeeding for women enrolled in the WIC program. This allows for women who are only practicing token breastfeeding to still be maintained on the program beyond the usual six weeks postpartum check-up period when they would be removed from the program in many states if they are formula feeding. WIC does allow expanded food packages for women who breastfeed exclusively and thus accept no formula vouchers.

An example of a follow-up record card that enables documentation to be kept on the exclusivity of breastfeeding is illustrated in Figure 1C-2. Computer databases can be established based on an intensity classification system that allows each patient's entry to reflect the total breast, water, formula, or other solid/vitamin feeding in any given 24-hour period. This will assist the clinician to draw conclusions about duration and health outcome by providing dose–response data.

In programs that encompass large geographic areas, the use of laptop computers and networking via computer to manage patient databases also allows for better communication among staff who are covering telephone warmlines and hotlines at sites removed from the patient and enables satellite areas to print documentation onto labels that can be entered into a centralized medical record.

Breastfeeding Follow-Up Record

Parents' Name: _____
Address: _____
Tele: _____ Infant's Birthday: _____ County: _____ Clinic Site # _____ M / F
Add. Phone: _____ Med. Info _____ Infant's Birthweight: _____ Medicaid #: _____
Hospital _____ S. S. # _____ Infant's Full Name: _____

	DELIVERY yes no	DISCHARGE yes no	1-3 DAYS yes no	5-7 DAYS yes no	10-12 DAYS yes no	1 MONTH yes no	6 WEEKS yes no	2 MONTHS yes no	3 MONTHS yes no							
DATE CONTACTED																
# FEEDINGS/24 HRS:																
FEEDING LENGTH (intervals between breastfeeding)																
ARTIFICIAL NIPPLES/ OTHER DEVICES																
EXPRESSION OF BREASTMILK School / Work/ Pump Loan																
TYPE, TIMING & AMOUNT OF OTHER FEEDINGS/VITAMINS																
BABY'S WEIGHT																
COMMENTS If Quit, Why?																
BREASTFEEDING STATUS DEFINITION																
FULL:																
EXCLUSIVE																
ALMOST EXCLUSIVE																
PARTIAL:																
HIGH																
MEDIUM																
LOW																
TOKEN																
DATE																

Lactation Consultant Project, GA Dept of Human Resources, District Six (6) WIC Program, June, 1993

Figure 1C-2 Front of breastfeeding follow-up record card maintained on each lactating woman in the East Central Health District, Augusta, Georgia.
Reprinted with permission.

Referred by: _____ Date: _____ On WIC: _____ YES or NO

Race: W B A I O   Marital Status: M S D Sep   Birthdate: _____ Age: _____

Have you BF before? _____ How long? _____ G ___ P ___ A ___ LC ___ Educ. Level of Mom _____ Dad _____

Does mother/father smoke? _____ YES or NO   Type of delivery: _____

	4 MONTHS yes no	5 MONTHS yes no	6 MONTHS yes no	7 MONTHS yes no	8 MONTHS yes no	9 MONTHS yes no	10 MONTHS yes no	11 MONTHS yes no	12 MONTHS yes no
DATE CONTACTED									
# FEEDINGS/24 HRS:									
FEEDING LENGTH (intervals between breastfeeding)									
ARTIFICIAL NIPPLES/ OTHER DEVICES									
EXPRESSION OF BREASTMILK School/Work/Pump Loan									
TYPE, TIMING & AMOUNT OF OTHER FEEDINGS/VITAMINS									
BABY'S WEIGHT									
COMMENTS If Quit, Why?									
BREASTFEEDING STATUS DEFINITION									
FULL:									
EXCLUSIVE									
ALMOST EXCLUSIVE									
PARTIAL:									
HIGH									
MEDIUM									
LOW									
TOKEN									
DATE									

Lactation Consultant Project, GA Dept of Human Resources, District Six (6) WIC Program, June, 1993

Figure 1C–2 continued Back of breastfeeding follow-up record card.

DETAILS ON FACTORS INFLUENCING DURATION

The National Surveys of Family Growth (NSFG) and the Ross Laboratories Mothers' Surveys (RLMS) (Ryan et al., 1991a) have reported breastfeeding rates for approximately thirty years. The NSFGs were collected by the National Center for Health Statistics in four cycles (1973, 1976, 1982, 1988) and data were collected in face-to-face interviews. The RLMS is a national mail survey designed to determine patterns of infant feeding during the first six months of life; the survey began in 1955 and continues annually. Similar rates of breastfeeding are reported by both surveys, with a decline in breastfeeding from 1955 to the early 1970s, followed by an upward trend until 1982 (Ryan et al., 1991a).

These similarities in rates of breastfeeding are evident across several maternal sociodemographic characteristics. The highest incidence of breastfeeding in the United States is reported among mothers with at least some college education, white or Hispanic ethnicity, having an infant of normal birthweight and increasing maternal age (Ryan et al., 1991b). Data from 1983 and 1984 show the lowest incidence of breastfeeding occurs among African Americans, those less than twenty years of age, at low income levels and among the less educated (Ryan et al., 1991a). Data from 1989 revealed that working, participating in WIC, and not living in the western United States also were risk factors for duration or lack of initiation of breastfeeding (Ryan et al., 1991b). A comparison of rates from 1984 to 1989 showed a decline in initiation of 13% (from 59.7% to 52.2%) and a decline in duration at six months (from 23.8% to 18.1%) (Ryan et al., 1991b). The decline in the rates of initiation in the less affluent was greater than the decline in the more affluent (Ryan et al., 1991b).

The influence of the hospital period on successful breastfeeding has been extensively studied. Hospital policies and practices, such as supplementing infants with formula (Marandi et al., 1993) and delaying the initiation of lactation (Kurinij & Shiono, 1991), have been reported to negatively influence breastfeeding duration, and the provision of formula discharge packs has been reported to alter duration and to negatively influence it (Bergevin et al., 1983; Gray-Donald et al., 1985). Stronger than information retained from verbal education discouraging the use of formula is the formula supplementation role model seen in the hospital (Snell et al., 1992). Dungy et al. (1992) showed that inclusion of a breast pump in and removal of formula from the discharge package increased duration of breastfeeding.

Breastfeeding support by professional staff educated in lactation management has been shown to positively impact breastfeeding duration (Auerbach, 1985; Johnson, Garza & Nichols, 1984; Jones & West, 1985; Macquart-Moulin et al., 1990). However, other studies have not demonstrated the same results (Grossman et al., 1990). Three of the four studies reporting a positive influence of hospital personnel on duration used an approach involving lactation professionals (Auerbach, 1985; Johnson, Garza & Nichols, 1984; Jones & West, 1985). In one study of 506 intervention patients and 151 controls, interventions aimed at providing information to women, supporting them after delivery, and raising the awareness of their environment coupled with educating health-care professionals were successful in increasing the number of women breastfeeding at one month (Kurinij & Shiono, 1991).

Grossman et al. (1990) investigated the effectiveness of intensive hospital-based postpartum support for low-income breastfeeding women by studying 97 women who were randomized to receive the usual support by obstetrical nurses or an intervention of education and extensive support by professionals educated in lactation management. No differences in duration were reported between the two groups. However, early introduction of formula and younger maternal age decreased duration, though participation in prenatal classes increased duration (Grossman et al., 1990).

Having an infant of normal birthweight (Ryan et al., 1991b) has been shown to be positively associated with breastfeeding for six months. The mother of an infant with a low birthweight is reported to be less likely to initiate breastfeeding or be breastfeeding at six months of age (Ryan et al., 1991b).

Posthospital discharge factors **negatively** influencing breastfeeding duration include the following:

- perceptions of insufficient milk supply (Forman et al., 1992; Kar & De, 1991; Pichaipat, et al., 1992)
- rigid feeding schedules (Lindenberg, Artola, & Estrada, 1990)
- supplementation with formula and other foods (Lindenberg, Artola & Estrada, 1990; Msuya et al., 1990; Perez-Escamilla et al., 1992; Retallack et al., 1994)
- aggressive marketing by infant foods companies undermining mother's confidence (Freed, 1993; Greiner, Van Esterick, & Latham, 1981)
- infant/mother sleep separation (Lindenberg, Aratola, & Estrada, 1990)
- nipple soreness or retraction (Salih et al., 1993)
- lack of social support or help to breastfeed (Forman et al., 1990)
- incompatibility of employment/child care with breastfeeding (Lindenberg, Artola, & Estrada, 1990; Pichaipat et al., 1992; Weile et al., 1990)
- lower socioeconomic status (Forman et al., 1990; Msuya et al., 1990; Perez-Escamilla et al., 1992; Retallack et al., 1994; Ryan et al., 1991b; Salih et al., 1993; Vestermark et al., 1991; Weile et al., 1990)

Factors **positively** impacting on breastfeeding duration include the following:

- ego maturity (Jacobson, Jacobson, & Frye, 1991)
- preparedness of mother—previous breastfeeding experience (Msuya et al., 1990; Perez-Escamilla et al., 1992; Perez-Gil-Romo et al., 1993)
- attendance at prenatal classes (Grossman et al., 1990)
- residence in a rural community in less developed countries (Perez-Escamilla, 1993; Salih et al., 1993)

In many parts of the world, the higher the socioeconomic class or education (Perez-Escamilla, 1993), the less likely the mother is to breastfeed for an extended duration, in contrast to most developed countries where the reverse is true (Ryan et al., 1991b). The degree of urbanization of the culture has been shown to negatively impact duration rates in developed countries (Lindenberg, Artola, & Estrada, 1990; Weile et al., 1990) and less developed countries (Perez-Escamilla, 1993). Strong cultural associations between breastfeeding incidence and ethnic background have been reported (Bryant, 1982; Entwisle, Doering, & Reilly, 1982; Rassin et al., 1984). In one study of breastfeeding initiation in a triethnic population, ethnicity was a determinant of the feeding method chosen only for Mexican Americans, although the odds of breastfeeding among Caucasians compared with African Americans depends on the level of maternal education (Bee et al., 1991).

Research exploring the relationship of acculturation into the United States to the initiation of breastfeeding suggest that women being assimilated into the United States are inhibited in the initiation of breastfeeding (Rassin et al., 1993). The relationship between ethnicity and duration is less clear, with some studies showing no relationship between duration and race (Grossman, 1990) or duration and lower socioeconomic level (Lindenberg, Artola, & Estrada, 1990; Weile et al., 1990) and others (Ryan et al., 1991b) reporting a positive association between ethnicity and duration.

The approaches to facilitate an increased incidence and extended duration of breastfeeding point to the need to consider the culture in which it is to be implemented. Also, important is the inclusion of educational curriculums for professionals and programs for the patients that include a breastfeeding component, support in the early postpartum period, and interventions addressing problems associated with milk-supply maintenance and maternal employment.

Community and Social Support

Social support is defined by Riordan (1989) as the subjective feelings of belonging, being accepted, and loved. When women who are breastfeeding feel they belong, are accepted, and loved, they tend to be more motivated to breastfeed longer. Social support can come from a variety of places: family support, peer support, organization support, and support by caregiving or helping professionals (Riordan, 1989).

The importance of family support appears to be influenced by culture and to be selective. Puerto Rican and Cuban women turn to their mothers for breastfeeding support and advice. Anglo women look to friends and husbands for support. For women of color, close friends and family members play a major role in the decision to breastfeed. Also, the mother's relationship with her parents tends to be perceived as more salient and positive than her relationship with her spouse's parents after the birth of the first child (Riordan, 1989).

Research suggests that if certain community-support mechanisms are in place women tend to breastfeed more and for longer periods of time. These mechanisms include, but are not limited to, individual counseling, peer-group discussions, postpartum support through hospital and clinics (Breastfeeding Clinic) and networking among health-care and social service workers who care for disadvantaged mothers and infants (Heiser, 1990; Selby, 1977). Breastfeeding outreach programs are using this research in the development of their programs.

BEST START, INC.

Best Start is an example of a breastfeeding-promotion program developed after 40 focus-group interviews were conducted to identify the common barriers to breastfeeding among women in the southeastern United States. The program is designed to reach the women least likely to breastfeed, including economically disadvantaged women in the United States. Common barriers to breastfeeding identified include lack of confidence, embarrassment, loss of freedom, dietary and health practices, and the influence of family and friends. A training manual and training tape is available for use when training counselors on how to address these barriers for women. The program encourages a three-step approach that will counteract the lack of confidence and lack of knowledge at the root of women's fears and doubts. The three steps include eliciting the mother's concerns, acknowledging her feelings, and educating her using carefully targeted messages. Best Start has produced many print and audiovisual materials based on the social marketing strategy to combine the principles and techniques of commercial marketing with more traditional health-education methods to promote a socially beneficial product, practice, or issue.

PUBLIC HEALTH—SPECIAL SUPPLEMENTAL NUTRITION PROGRAM FOR WOMEN, INFANTS AND CHILDREN

The Special Supplemental Nutrition Program for Women, Infants and Children (WIC) was instituted in 1972 by the U.S. Department of Agriculture. The purpose of the WIC program is to provide low-income women and children who are at risk for medical or nutritional problems with certain nutritious supplemental foods, nutrition education, and access to other health-care programs. The goal of WIC is to prevent health problems during critical periods of growth and development.

WIC services are available in every state and territory. Each state agency and Native American tribe creates its own food package, nutrition education component, qualifying risk factors, and administrative details based on its populations' needs and funded money. Guidelines for Breastfeeding Promotion and Support in the WIC program were last revised in 1993 by the National Association of WIC Directors (NAWD) Breastfeeding Promotion Committee. Final regulations on the requirements for breastfeeding promotion and support activities in the WIC program were published in the *Federal Register* (59:48, 11503 to 11504) on March 11, 1994.

The final regulations delineate the following state and local agency requirements:

1. Provide training on the promotion and management of breastfeeding to staff at local agencies who will provide information and assistance to participants.
2. Identify or develop resources and educational materials, which are culturally and educationally appropriate, for use in local agencies.
3. Document and evaluate breastfeeding promotion and support activities annually, including participants' views of the local program's effectiveness. Monitor local agency activities to ensure compliance with the following:
   - Policies and practices that create a positive clinic environment.
   - Designation by each local agency of a staff person to coordinate breastfeeding promotion and support activities.
   - Incorporation by each local agency of task-appropriate training into orientation programs for new staff involved in direct contact with WIC clients.
   - A plan to ensure that women have access to breastfeeding promotion and support activities during the prenatal and postpartum periods.

The local agency is responsible for all the items listed under number 3; the state agency evaluates the local agency's performance.

Active breastfeeding promotion is ongoing among many WIC programs. Some WIC districts have developed programs that utilize peer and professional counselors in an effort to promote and support breastfeeding. Postpartum practices designed to support breastfeeding in WIC populations include telephone, home, and clinic visits; telephone warm (limited access) and hot (24-hour access) lines; pump programs, prenatal classes, and support groups (U.S. Department of Agriculture, Food and Nutrition Service, 1988).

LA LECHE LEAGUE INTERNATIONAL

La Leche League International (LLLI) is a nonsectarian, not-for-profit educational and service organization incorporated in the state of Illinois. It was founded in Franklin Park, a suburb of Chicago, in 1956. Seven women came together during a time when artificial feeding was rapidly replacing breastfeeding as the preferred

Table 1C–1   La Leche League Meeting Topics

1. The Advantage of Breastfeeding to Mother, Baby and Family
2. The Baby Arrives: The Breastfed Baby and the Family
3. The Art of Breastfeeding and Overcoming Difficulties
4. Nutrition and Weaning

infant-feeding choice in a progressive society. Today La Leche League reaches more than 100,000 mothers in more than 46 countries. The heart of La Leche League is a "mother-to-mother" support system. Volunteer group leaders are trained and experienced breastfeeding mothers who are also familiar with current research. They offer practical information and ongoing support to nursing mothers through monthly meetings and telephone help.

The La Leche League is a community-based organization headed by a local leader. The type of support provided by La Leche League, a combination of practical information and personal caring, has been shown to substantially increase a mother's chances of succeeding in breastfeeding her baby. It is noteworthy that LLLI is the world's largest resource for breastfeeding information, publishing 20 books, information sheets, pamphlets, in addition to a bimonthly periodical for breastfeeding women. A newsletter for health-care professionals is published quarterly.

La Leche League maintains a health advisory council of 43 health professionals who are consulted on medical issues and review current research. The annual physicians' seminars offer continuing medical education credits to health-care professionals. Although LLLI meetings are widely accepted as offering support only, they can provide a unique opportunity for women to experience the many dimensions of breastfeeding first-hand. Monthly, guided group discussions are held following a rotating topic outline based on the League's 1991 manual, *The Womanly Art of Breastfeeding* (see Table 1C–1). These monthly meetings provide a means for seasoned breastfeeding mothers, acting as group leaders, to teach the art of breastfeeding through discussion, information, and mother-to-mother sharing.

Contact with LLLI mimics the traditional way breastfeeding and other functions of motherhood (i.e., childbirth, mothering) were disseminated in any given culture. Some LLLI groups offer special meetings that focus on concerns of mothers with nursing toddlers or that include fathers and address topics specific to mothers and fathers of breastfeeding infants. When a class format combines practical information with sound adult learning techniques, chances for a positive impact on breastfeeding success, perceived and real, are increased.

PEER-COUNSELOR PROGRAMS

Peer-counseling programs help mothers know that they can breastfeed by instilling confidence. Many mothers believe that breastfeeding is instinctive and therefore may be reluctant to seek help if they encounter problems. Peer counselors provide support systems within the community that will provide ongoing information and help services. Many county health department offices have adopted peer-counselor programs to encourage and support mothers who are breastfeeding. The counseling that experienced breastfeeding mothers provide can serve to eliminate fears and inhibitions. Where peer counselors are in place, breastfeeding rates have been reported to increase dramatically. The Interagency Group for Breastfeeding Promotion states that a breastfeeding-promotion program needs mother-to-mother support as well as professional training to be sustainable and have maximum effect.

La Leche League International's Peer Counselor Program can serve as a model. The program pairs experienced and trained LLLI leaders with economically disadvantaged women who have breastfed their babies and trains them as peer counselors. The 25-hour training program provides the peer counselor with the skills and information to give breastfeeding presentations at clinics, work one-to-one with mothers, lead support groups, and provide telephone help for women with breastfeeding problems. The training encourages mother-to-mother sharing, which helps the trainees feel more secure with their role as breastfeeding mothers and as peer support leaders.

Local and state public health departments and WIC programs have designed training formats for peer-counselor programs. Peer-support programs for post-partum follow-up have grown in popularity in the WIC program, although limited data on the efficiency of peer support instead of professional support exists. Kistin et al. (1994) evaluated the effect of peer counselors on breastfeeding initiation, exclusivity, and duration among low-income urban women in the midwestern United States. The study compared the infant-feeding practices of women who planned to breastfeed and received support from counselors to women who requested counselors but did not receive support because of a lack of personnel. Women assigned counselors prenatally had a significantly ($p < .05$) higher breast-feeding-initiation rate—93% verses 70%—than the no-counselor group of women. Exclusivity and duration were also significantly higher ($p < .05$) in the counselor group. Among women in the counselor group, 64% breastfed longer than 6 weeks and 44% longer than 12 weeks compared with the no-counselor groups—28% and 21%, respectively. The mean number of weeks of any breastfeeding in the counselor group was 15 weeks, in contrast to a mean of 8 weeks in the no-counselor group ($p < .05$). In this study, counselors did not document every call or contact and, thus, an assessment of a dose–response effect of the counselors was not possible (Kistin et al., 1994).

In a study of 97 women enrolled in WIC in which follow-up was randomized to a peer (P) or a professional (PROF) and there were no significant differences in maternal age, ethnicity, or education, infant birthweight or gestational age, the difference in duration of breastfeeding was not significant. Of the 97 women, 21 were lost to follow-up (12 P, 9 PROF) 65 women quit breastfeeding before six months (28/44 P, 37/53 PROF), and 11 breastfed beyond six months (4/44 vs. 7/53) (Black, Davis, & Bhatia, 1995). Although this study suggests that peer support in this population resulted in similar duration of breastfeeding than that of professional support, it cannot be conclusively stated because of the large percentage of patients lost to follow-up and small sample size that reached six months of breastfeeding.

BREASTFEEDING EDUCATORS

Breastfeeding educators are individuals who assess, plan, intervene, and evaluate normal breastfeeding relationships. Usually they have other clinical responsibilities and provide their service as part of an institution/organization. They may hold certification by a community or regional agency. All professionals working in maternal and child health areas should be skilled at the level of a breastfeeding educator so they can assist families in initiating breastfeeding and understanding the process of lactation. Breastfeeding educators make referrals to lactation consultants in more specialized situations or for complex problems.

LACTATION CONSULTANTS

Recent strides have been made in recognizing the need for the benefits offered by the lactation consultant. The role of the lactation consultant continues to be defined. The primary focus of the consultant is as a clinical specialist to assist in problematic complex situations or offer expertise regarding special circumstances to the primary caregiver.

Lactation consultants come from a variety of backgrounds, including dietitians, registered nurses, WIC nutritionists, midwives, La Leche League leaders, and physicians. Lactation consultants have an official certifying organization, the International Board of Certifying Lactation Consultant Examiners (IBCLE).

The International Lactation Consultant Association (ILCA) is the official professional organization of the lactation consultant. Lactation consultants are found in a variety of settings, including hospitals, private practice, corporate practice, public health practice, and academic/research practice.

Families who need specialized breastfeeding assistance benefit from an early referral to a consultant. A physician, health professional, or self referral to a lactation consultant is appropriate (for suggestions on when to refer to a lactation consultant, see Table 1C–2). Once a referral is received, the lactation consultant meets with the family to identify their concerns and collaborates with the physician and health-care team. A plan to assist each family to meet their breastfeeding goals is developed, implemented, and revised as necessary. Follow-up is continued until the problem is resolved.

The duties and qualifications of lactation consultants and how referrals are received varies according to the setting in which he or she practices. For legal protection, maintaining malpractice insurance and obtaining informed consent prior to assisting a breastfeeding mother and baby are two issues that those working in lactation should address.

WELL START INTERNATIONAL

Well Start is a training program designed to train teams of health-care professionals in lactation management. Teams from throughout the United States and around the world have been trained by this California-based program. Teams include representatives from the medical, nursing, nutrition, and lactation professions.

Table 1C–2   Suggestions for Referrals to Lactation Consultants

- Mother is very anxious about breastfeeding—especially if breastfeeding a previous infant was not a positive experience
- Mother has flat or inverted nipples
- Latch-on and/or audible swallowing has not occurred by 24 hours after birth
- Infant has difficulty breastfeeding
- Latch-on and swallowing not consistent
- Feeding lasts > one hour
- Infant is hungry after most feedings
- Mother is experiencing unrelieved pathologic engorgement
- Mother and infant separated during hospitalization
- Mother has cracked or blistered nipples or nipple soreness has not improved by five days after birth
- Infant had inadequate output: <2 bowel movements or <6 urinations in 24 hours in neonatal period
- Infant has inadequate weight gain or has not regained birthweight by two weeks of age
- Infant displays signs of suck (nipple) confusion—accepts bottle but not breast
- Actual or perceived low milk supply
- Infant or mother has specific medical condition that may interfere with initiating or maintaining lactation

Legal Issues Surrounding Breastfeeding

The incidence and duration of breastfeeding is the United States has increased over the last century. With this increased incidence, there is also an increased number of legal cases involving breastfeeding mothers. Social and legal institutions that are part of everyday life in the United States do not always reflect the changing attitudes about breastfeeding that have led to increased incidence of breastfeeding. Breastfeeding conflicts with social customs, business rules and regulations, county ordinances, and court orders. These conflicts are being resolved through litigation and calls for changes in ordinances, rules, and regulations:

1977:   A New York mother, nursing discreetly and covered by a large beach towel, was watching her older children swim in a community pool. Management prohibited her from breastfeeding. The mother sued and won (Lofton & Gotsch, 1983).

1981:   An Iowa mother was asked to stop nursing her infant in a family restaurant. The mother filed a complaint with the local Human Rights Commission. The restaurant chain later agreed to allow mothers to nurse in their restaurants (Lofton & Gotsch, 1983).

1981:   A Missouri mother was warned by a police officer not to breastfeed in a parked car in the shopping center parking lot or risk being cited for indecent exposure. The mother contacted a county councilwoman, who proposed a new ordinance allowing mothers to breastfeed in public. The council agreed and the existing county ordinance on indecent exposure was rewritten to exclude breastfeeding (Lofton & Gotsch, 1983).

1981:   One of the most influential cases is the *Dike* case. Janice Dike, a kindergarten teacher, sued Orange County, Florida, for prohibiting her from breastfeeding on school grounds. The Fifth U.S. Circuit Court of Appeals ruled in Mrs. Dike's favor, stating: "Breastfeeding is the most elemental form of parental care. It is a communion between mother and child that, like marriage is 'intimate to the degree of being sacred'. . . . We conclude that the Constitution protects from excessive state interference a woman's decision respecting breastfeeding her child" (*The Washington Post*, 1981).

1984:   New York amends its indecent-exposure law to exempt breastfeeding.

1993:   The Florida legislature amended the state's statutes on indecent exposure to exempt and protect nursing mothers from arrest or harassment by law-enforcement or private security officials. The bill condemns "the vicious cycle of embarrassment and ignorance" and "archaic and outdated moral taboos" surrounding the practice, endorsing breastfeeding instead as the preferred method of nurturing an infant (Rohter, 1993).

The Family and Medical Leave Act (FMLA) of 1993 entitles employees to take up to 12 weeks of unpaid, job-protected leave each year for specified family and medical reasons. The FMLA requires employers who have 50 or more employees to participate. Employees are eligible if they have worked for a covered employer for at least one year and for 1,250 hours during the previous 12 months.

1994:   Legislators in New York passed a civil rights measure to protect breastfeeding women from being harassed if nursing their babies in public. The law imposes fines of up to $5,000 or a prison sentence of up to five years for those who try to prevent them from nursing.

Other legal issues related to breastfeeding, including jury duty exemption, jailed mothers, and divorce/custody/visitation battles, are still being deliberated. The maternity leave issue was addressed in the Pregnancy Disability Act (October 1978), which called for employers to provide insurance and disability coverage for pregnancy on the same basis as for any other medical condition (Lofton & Gotsch, 1983). The FMLA lengthens by four to six weeks the usual maternity leave for those women who are employed by companies that are required to comply. Still, there are many legal issues to be addressed before breastfeeding again becomes the norm.

POST-TEST

For questions 1 to 4, choose the best answer.

1. Extended duration of breastfeeding is important because
   A. the mother's menstrual cycle will not return unless breastfeeding is exclusive.
   B. the continued production of breastmilk depends on it.
   C. health benefits increase with increased "doses" of breastmilk.
   D. milk constituents that confer immunity are not present until after several months of breastfeeding.

2. Breastfeeding for less than 75% but more than 25% of feedings is considered
   A. token breastfeeding.
   B. high-partial breastfeeding.
   C. full breastfeeding.
   D. medium-partial breastfeeding.

3. Breastfeeding in a manner that no liquid or solid other than breastmilk, water, and/or vitamins/minerals is given to the infant is best described as
   A. high-partial breastfeeding.
   B. exclusive breastfeeding.
   C. almost exclusive breastfeeding.
   D. medium-partial breastfeeding.

4. Token breastfeeding is defined as
   A. more than 80% of feeds are breastmilk.
   B. feeding no liquid or solid other than breastmilk to the infant.
   C. breastfeeding episodes that have insignificant caloric contribution.
   D. 20% to 79% of feeds are breastmilk.

For questions 5 to 10, choose the best answer from the following key:
   A. Positively associated with long duration of breastfeeding
   B. Negatively associated with long duration of breastfeeding

5. Normal birthweight

6. Incompatibility of employment with breastfeeding

7. Maternal ego maturity

8. Previous breastfeeding experience

9. Rigid feeding schedule

10. Supplementation with formula and other foods

For questions 11 to 15, choose the best answer from the following key:
   A. **Best Start**
   B. **Special Supplemental Nutrition Program for Women, Infants and Children**
   C. **La Leche League International**
   D. **International Board of Lactation Consultant Examiners**
   E. **International Lactation Consultant Association**

11. Services include nutrition and breastfeeding education combined with food vouchers

12. Social marketing approach to reach low-income women through the print and visual media

13. Founded in 1956 by seven breastfeeding mothers

14. Certifies lactation consultants

15. Professional organization for lactation consultants

For questions 16 and 17, choose the best answer from the following key:
   A. **New York**
   B. **Florida**

16. State that first amended its indecent-exposure law to exempt breastfeeding women and 10 years later passed a civil rights measure to protect breastfeeding women from being harassed in public.

17. First state to protect nursing mothers from arrest or harassment by law-enforcement or private security officials.

For questions 18 to 20, choose the best answer from the following key:
   A. **Peer counselors**
   B. **Lactation consultants**
   C. **Breastfeeding educators**

18. Provide mother-to-mother support

19. Handle complex breastfeeding situations

20. Provide basic breastfeeding assistance in the health-care environment

References

Abbey, LM (1979). Is breast feeding a likely cause of dental caries in young children? *J Am Dent Assoc*, 98: 21-23.

Amador, M, Hermelo, MP, Canetti, JE, Consuegra, E (1992). Adolescent mothers: Do they breast-feed less? *Acta Paediatr Hung*, 32(3):269-85.

Ameda Egnell (1991). Ten myths about breastfeeding. *Circle of Caring*, 4(3):1.

Auerbach, KG (1985). The influence of lactation consultant contact on breastfeeding duration in a low-income population. *Neb Med J*, 70:341-46.

Auerbach, KG (1990a). Assisting the employed breast-feeding mother. *J Nurse-Midwifery*, 35(1):26-34.

Auerbach, KG (1990b). Breastfeeding fallacies: Their relationship to understanding lactation. *Birth*, 17(1):44-48.

Auerbach, KG, Guss, E (1984). Maternal employment and breastfeeding: A study of 567 women's experiences. *Am J Dis Child*, 138(10):958-60.

Backas, N (1996). Breastfeeding in Canada. *Rental Roundup*, 13(2):4-5.

Balsamo, F, De Mari, G, Maher, V, Serini, R (1992). Production and pleasure: Research on breast-feeding in Turin. In: Maher, V, *The Anthropology of Breast-Feeding*, Berg: Oxford, 59-90.

Baranowski, T, Bee, DE, Rassin, DK, Richardson, CJ, Brown, JP, Guenther, N, Nader, PR (1983). Social support, social influence, ethnicity and the breastfeeding decision. *Soc Sci Med*, 17(21):1599-1611.

Baranowski, T, Rassin, DK, Richardson, CJ, Brown, JP, Bee, DE (1986). Attitudes toward breastfeeding. *J Dev Behav Pediatr*, 7(6):367-72.

Baumslag, N, Putney, P (Eds.) (1989). Breastfeeding: *The Passport to Life*. NGO Committee on UNICEF: New York.

Becerra, JE, Smith, JC (1990). Breastfeeding patterns in Puerto Rico. *Am J Public Health*, 80(6):694-97.

Bee, D, et al. (1991). Breastfeeding initiation in a triethnic population. *Am J Dis Child*, 145:306-9.

Bergevin, Y, Dougherty, C, Kramer, SM (1983). Do formula samples shorten the duration of breastfeeding? *Lancet*, 1:1148.

Bernshaw, NB (1992). Teaching breastfeeding through the myths. *Rental Roundup*, 2(9):2-3.

Bevan, ML, Mosley, D, Lobach, KS, Solimano, GR (1984). Factors influencing breastfeeding in an urban WIC program. *J Am Diet Assoc*, 84:563.

Birenbaum, E, Vila, Y, Linder, N, Reichman, B (1993). Continuation of breast-feeding in an Israeli population. *J Pediatr Gastroenterol Nutr*, 16(3):311-15.

Black, RF, Blair, JP, Jones, VN, DuRant, RH (1990). Infant feeding decisions among pregnant women from a WIC population in Georgia. *J Am Diet Assoc*, 90(2):255-59.

Black, RF, Davis, H, Bhatia, J (1995). Breastfeeding in a low income population: Effect of peer or professional lactational support. *Pediatr Res*, 37(4), Part 2:250A, Abstract 1488.

Brogan, BD, Fox, HM (1984). Infant feeding practices of low- and middle-income families in Nebraska. *J Am Diet Assoc*, 84:560-63.

Bryant, CA (1982). The impact of kin, friend and neighbor networks on infant feeding practices. *Soc Sci Med*, 16:1757-65.

Bryant, CA, Roy, M (1990). *Best Start Training Manual: Breastfeeding for healthy mothers, healthy babies*. Best Start, Inc.: Tampa.

Bureau of Census (1992). Statistical Abstract of the United States, p. 385. Washington, DC: US Department of Commerce.

Bureau of National Affairs Special Report (1986). *Work and the Family: A Changing Dynamic*, p. 13. Washington, DC: Bureau of National Affairs.

Chandra, RK (1979). Prospective studies of the effect of breastfeeding on incidence of infection and allergy. *Acta Paediatr Scand*, 68:691-94.

Chandra, RK (1992). Food allergy: 1992 and beyond. *Nutr Res*, 12:93-99.

Chia, SF (1992). A survey of breast feeding practices in infants seen in general practice. *Med J Malaysia*, 47(2):134-38.

Chung, MH, Chung, KK, Chung, CS, Raymond, JS (1992-1993). Health-related behaviors in Korea: Smoking, drinking, prenatal care. *Asia Pac J Public Health*, 6(1):10-15.

Cochi, S, Fleming, D, et al. (1986). Primary invasive Haemophilus influenza type b disease: a population-based assessment of risk factor. *Pediatrics*, 108:887-96

Cohen, R., Mrtek, MB (1994). The impact of two corporate lactation programs on the incidence and duration of breastfeeding by employed mothers. *Am J Health Promot*, 8(6):436-41.

Creyghton, ML (1992). Breast-feeding and Baraka in Northern Tunisia. In: Maher, V. *The Anthropology of Breast-Feeding*. Berg: Oxford, pp. 37-58.

Dana, N, Price, A (1987). *The Working Woman's Guide to Breastfeeding*. Meadowbrook: New York.

Drucker, P (1974). *Management*. Harper & Row: New York, p. 61.

Duffy, LC, Riepenoff-Talty, M, Ogra, P, et al. (1986). Modulation of rotavirus enteritis during breastfeeding. *Am J Dis Child*, 140:1164-68.

Duncan, B, Ey, J, Holberg, CJ, et al. (1993). Exclusive breastfeeding for at least four months protects against otitis media. *Pediatrics*, 91:867-72

Dungy, CI, Christensen-Szalanski, J, Losch, M, Russell, D (1992). Effect of discharge samples of duration of breast-feeding. *Pediatrics*, 90(2):233-37.

Entwisle, RR, Doering, SG, Reilly, TW (1982). Sociopsychological determinants of women's breastfeeding behavior. A replication and extension. *Am J Orthopsychiatry*, 52:244.

Fallot, ME, Boyd, JL, Oski, FA (1980). Breastfeeding reduces incidence of hospital admissions for infections in infants. *Pediatrics*, 65:1121-24.

Forman, MR, Hundt, GL, Towne, D, Graubard, B, Sullivan, B, Berendes, HW, Saarov, B, Naggan, L (1990). The forty-day rest period and infant feeding practices among Negev Bedouin Arab women in Israel. *Medical Anthropol*, 12(2):207-16.

Forman, MR, Hundt, GL, Graubard, BI, Chang, D, Sarov, B, Naggan, L, Berendes, HW (1992). Factors influencing milk insufficiency and its long-term health effects: The Bedouin Infant Feeding Study. *Int J Epidemiol*, 21(1):53-58.

Frederickson, D (1994). Lecture, International Lactation Consultant Association Annual Meeting, Atlanta.

Freed, GL (1993). Breast-feeding: Time to teach what we preach. *JAMA*, 269(2):243-45.

Freed, GL, Fraley, JK, Schanler, RJ (1992). Attitudes of expectant fathers regarding breast-feeding. *Pediatrics*, 90(2 Pt 1):224-27.

Gabriel, A, Gabriel, KR, Lawrence, RA (1986). Cultural value and biomedical knowledge: Choices in infant feeding. *Soc Sci Med*, 23:501.

Giugliani, ERJ, Caiaffa, WT, Vogelhut, J, Witter, FR, Perman, JA (1994). Effect of breastfeeding support from different sources on mothers' decisions to breastfeed. *J Hum Lact*, 10(3):157-61.

Gomez, DH, Garnica, ME, Sepulveda, J, Valdespino-Gomez, JL, Lam, N, Herrera, MC (1990). Lactation and weaning patterns in Mexico. 1986 National Health Survey corrected and republished with original paging; article originally printed *in Salud Publica Mex*, 1989 Nov–Dec, 31(6):725-34.

Grams, M (1985). *Breastfeeding Success for Working Mothers*. Achievement Press: Carson City, NV.

Gray-Donald, K, Kramer, MS, Munday, S, Leduc, DG (1985). Effect of formula supplementation in hospital on the duration of breastfeeding: A controlled clinical trial. *Pediatrics*, 75(3):514-18.

Greiner, T, Van Esterick, P, Latham, MC (1981). The insufficient milk syndrome: An alternative explanation. *Med Anthropol*, 5(232):233-60.

Grossman, LK, Harter, C, Sachs, L, Kay, JA (1990). The effect of postpartum lactation counseling on the duration of breastfeeding in low-income women. *Am J Dis Child*, 144(4):471-74.

Gunnlaugsson, G, Einarsd'ottr, J (1993). Colostrum and ideas about bad milk: A case study from Guinea-Bissau. *Soc Sci Med*, 36(3):283-88.

Harris, MC, Kolski, GB, Campbell, DE, et al. (1989). Ontogeny of the antibody response to cow milk proteins. *Ann Allergy*, 63:439-42.

Hastrup, K (1992). A question of reason: Breastfeeding patterns in seventeenth and eighteenth century. In: Maher, V, *The Anthropology of Breastfeeding* (pp. 91-108). Berg: Oxford.

Heiser, B (1990). Reaching out to all. *Breastfeeding Abs*, 9(4):19-20.

Heldenberg, D, Tenenbaum, Gl, Weizer, S (1993). Breastfeeding habits among Jewish and Arab mothers in Hadera County, Israel. *J Pediatr Gastroenterol Nutr*, 17(1): 86-91.

Helsing, E (1989). Nutrition policies in Europe—the state of the art. *Eur J Clin Nutr*, 43 Suppl (2):57-66.

Howie, PW, Forsyth, JS, Ogston, SA, et al. (1990). Protective effects of breastfeeding against infection. *Br Med J*, 300(6716):11-16.

Hundt, GL, Forman, MR (1993). Interfacing anthropology and epidemiology: The Bedouin Arab Infant Feeding Study. *Soc Sci Med*, 36(7):957-64.

Hunkeler, B, Aebi, C, Minder, CE, Bossi, E (1994). Incidence and duration of breastfeeding of ill newborns. *J Pediatr Gastroenterol Nutr*, 18(1):37-40.

Imperiale, N (1993). Nursing mothers in the workplace. *Orlando Sentinel*, E1-E4.

Jacobson, SW, Jacobson, JL, Frye, KF (1991). Incidence and correlates of breastfeeding in socioeconomically disadvantaged women. *Pediatrics*, 88(4):728-36.

Joesoef, MR, et al. (1989). A recent increase of breastfeeding duration in Jakarta, Indonesia. *Am J Public Health*, 79:36-38.

Johnson, CA, Garza C, Nichols, B (1984). A teaching intervention to improve breastfeeding success. *J Nutr Educ*, 16:19-22.

Jones, DA, West, RR (1985). Lactation nurses increase duration of breastfeeding. *Arch Dis Child*, 60:772-74.

Jordan, PL, Wall, VR (1993). Supporting the father when an infant is breastfed. *J Hum Lact*, 9(1):31-34.

Kaplowitz, DD, Olson, CM (1983). The effects of an education program on the decision to breastfeed. *J Nutr Educ*, 15(2):61-65.

Kar, M, De, R (1991). Breastfeeding practices—impressions from an urban community. *Indian J Public Health*, 35(4):93-96.

Karjalainen, J, Martin JM, Karp M, et al. (1992). A bovine albumin peptide as a possible trigger of insulin-dependent diabetes mellitus. *N Engl J Med*, 327:302-7.

Khatib-Chahidi, J (1992). Milk kinship in Shi'ite Islamic Iran. In: Maher, V, *The Anthropology of Breast-Feeding* (pp. 109-32). Berg: Oxford.

Kistin, N, Abramson, R, Dublin, P (1994). Effect of peer counselors on breastfeeding initation, exclusivity, duration among low-income urban women. *J Hum Lact*, 10(1):11-15.

Kitzinger, S (1987). *The Experience of Breastfeeding*. Penguin Books: New York.

Kocturk T, Zetterstrom, R (1989). The promotion of breastfeeding and maternal attitudes. *Acta Paediatr Scand*, 78:817-23.

Kurinij, N, Shiono, PH (1991). Early formula supplementation of breast-feeding. *Pediatrics*, 88(4):745-50.

La Leche League International (LLLI) (1991). *The Womanly Art of Breastfeeding*. LLLI: Franklin Park, IL.

Labbok, M, Krasovec, K (1990). Toward consistency in breastfeeding definitions. *Stud Fam Plann*, 21(4):226-30.

Larsson, E, Ogaard B, Lindsten, R (1993). Rearing of Swedish, Norwegian, and Norwegian Sami children. *Scand J Dent Res*, 101(6):382-85.

Laufer, AB (1990). Breastfeeding: Toward resolution of the unsatisfying birth experience. *J Nurse Midwifery*, 35(1): 42-45.

Lawrence, RA (1989). *Breastfeeding: A Guide for the Medical Profession*. Mosby: St. Louis.

Lawrence, RA (1994). *Breastfeeding: A Guide for the Medical Profession* (pp. 1-35). Mosby: St. Louis.

Leventhal, JM, et al. (1986). Does breastfeeding protect against infections in infants less than 3 months of age? *Pediatrics*, 78:896-903.

Lindenberg, CS, Artola, RC, Estrada, VJ (1990). Determinants of early infant weaning: A multivariate approach. *Int J Nurs Stud*, 27(10):35-41.

Littman, H, Medendorp, SV, Goldfarb, E (1994). The decision to breastfeed: The importance of fathers' approval. *Clin Pediatr*, 33:214-19.

Lizarraga, JL, Maehr, JC, Wingard, DL, Felice, ME (1992). Psychosocial and economic factors associated with infant feeding intentions of adolescent mothers. *J Adolesc Health*, 13(8):676-81.

Lofton, H, Gotsch, G (1983). Legal rights of breastfeeding mothers: USA scene. *Adv Int Matern Child Health*, 3.

Macquart-Moulin, G, Fancello, G, Vincent, A, Julin, C, Baret, C, Ayme, S (1990). Evaluation of the effects of a support campaign on exclusive breastfeeding at 1 month. *Revue D'Epidemiologie et de Santa Publique*, 38(3):201-9.

Magid, K, McKelvey, C (1987). *High Risk: Children Without a Conscience* (p. 248). Bantam Books: New York.

Maher, V (Ed.) (1992). *The Anthropology of Breastfeeding—Natural Law or Social Construct*. Berg: Oxford.

Marandi, A, Afzali, HM, Hossaini, AF (1993). The reasons for early weaning among mothers in Teheran. *Bull WHO*, 71(5):561-69.

Martinez, GA, Dodd, DA, Samartgedes, JA (1981). Milk feeding patterns in the United States during the first twelve months of life. *Pediatrics*, 68(6):863-68.

Martinez, GA, Nalezienski, JP (1981). 1980 update: The recent trend in breast-feeding. *Pediatrics*, 67(2):260-63.

Matich, JR, Sims, LS (1992). A comparison of social support variables between women who intend to breast or bottle feed. *Soc Sci Med*, 34:919-27.

Mayer, EJ, Hamman, RF, Gay, EC, et al. (1988). Reduced risk of IDDM among breast-fed children. *Diabetes*, 37: 1625-32.

McNatt, MH, Freston, MS (1992). Social support and lactation outcomes in postpartum women. *J Hum Lact*, 8(20):73-77.

Meftuh, AB, Tapsoba, LP, Lamounier, JA (1991). Breastfeeding practices in Ethiopian women in southern California. *Indian J Pediatr*, 58(3):349-56.

Merrett, TG, Burr, ML, Butland, BK, et al. (1988). Infant feeding and allergy: Twelve-month prospective study of 500 babies born in allergic families. *Ann Allergy*, 61(6 Pt 2):13-20.

Monteiro, C, et al. (1988). Breast-feeding patterns and socioeconomic status in the city of Sao Paulo. *J Trop Pediatr*, 34:186-92.

Msuya, JM, Harding, WR, Robinson, MF, McKenzie-Parnell, J (1990). The extent of breastfeeding in Dunedin 1974–83. *NZ Med J*, 103(884):68-70.

News Wave (1993). *Mother-Friendly Workplaces Mean Healthier Babies, Less Absenteeism*, Independence, WI, Sept. 2.

Newton, E (1992). Breastfeeding/lactation and the medical school curriculum. *J Hum Lact*, 8(3):122-24.

Newton, N (1971). Psychologic differences between breast and bottle feeding. In: Jelliffee, D, Jelliffe, EFP (Eds.), Symposium: The uniqueness of human milk. *Am J Clin Nutr*, 24:993.

Newton, N, Newton, M (1967). Psychologic aspects of lactation. *N Engl J Med*, 277(22):1179-88.

Novotny, R, Kieffer, EC, Mor, J, Thiele, M, Nikaido, M (1994). Health of infants is the main reason for breastfeeding in a WIC population in Hawaii. *J Am Diet Assoc*, 94(3): 293-97.

Palmer G (1988). *The Politics of Breastfeeding*. Pandora Press: London.

Palti, H, et al. (1984). Episodes of illness in breast-fed and bottle-fed infants in Jerusalem. *Israel J Med Sci*, 20:395-99.

Panter-Brick, C (1992). Working mothers in rural Nepal. In: Maher, V, *The Anthropology of Breastfeeding* (pp. 133-50). Berg: Oxford.

Pascoe, JM, Berger, A (1985). Attitudes of high school girls in Israel and the United States toward breastfeeding. *J Adolesc Health Care*, 6(1):28-30.

Perez-Escamilla, R (1993). Breastfeeding patterns in nine Latin American and Caribbean countries. *Bull Pan Am Health Organ*, 27(1):32-42.

Perez-Escamilla, R, Roman Perez, R, Mejia, LA, Dewey, KG (1992). Infant feeding practices among low-income Mexican urban women: A four-month follow-up. *Archivos Latinoamericanos de Nutricion*, 42(3):259-67.

Perez-Gil-Romo, SE, Rueda-Arroniz, F, Diez-Urdanivia-Coria, S (1993). Breastfeeding and child care: A case study of 2 rural areas of Mexico. *Salud Publica Mex*, 35(6):692-99.

Pichaipat, V, Thanomsingh, P, Pudhapongsiriporn, S, Buranasin, P, Pharidanunt, M, Monkalasiri, R (1992). An intervention model for breastfeeding in Maharat Nakhon Ratchasima Hospital. *Southeast Asian J Trop Med Public Health*, 23(3):439-43.

Popkin, BM, Canahuati, J, Bailey, PE, O'Gara, C (1991). An evaluation of a national breast-feeding promotion programme in Honduras. *J Biosoc Sci*, 23(1):5-21.

Pullan, CR, Toms, GL, Martin, AJ, et al. (1980). Breastfeeding and respiratory syncytial virus infection. *Br Med J*, 281(6247):1034-36.

Rassin, DK, Markides, KS, Baranowski, T, Bee, DE, Richardson, CJ, Mikrut, WD, Winkler, BA (1993). Acculturation and breastfeeding on the United States–Mexico border. *Am J Med Sci*, 306(1):28-34.

Rassin, DK, Richardson, CJ, Baranowski, T, Nader, PR, Guenther, N, Bee, DE, Brown, JP (1984). Incidence of breastfeeding in low socioeconomic group of mothers in the United States: Ethnic patterns. *Pediatrics*, 73(2):132-37.

Rassin, DK, Richardson, CJ, Baranowski, T (1986). Ethnic determinants of lactation in a population of mothers in the United States. *J Hum Lact*, 2:69-81.

Retallack, SJ, Simmer, K, Makrides, M, Gibson, RA (1994). Infant weaning practices in Adelaide: The results of a shopping complex survey. *J Paediatr Child Health*, 30(1):28-32.

Riordan, J (1989). Social support and breastfeeding. *Breastfeeding Abst*, 8(3):13-14.

Riordan, J, Auerbach, K (1993). *Breastfeeding and Human Lactation*. Jones and Bartlett: Boston.

Rohter, L (1993). Florida approves measure on right to breastfeed in public. *The New York Times*, March 4.

Ross (1986-1995). *Annual Infant Feeding Survey*. Ross Products Division, Abbott Laboratories: Columbus, OH.

Ryan, AS, Martinez, GA (1989). Breastfeeding and the working mother: A profile. *Pediatrics*, 83(4):524-31.

Ryan, AS, Prapp, WF, Wysong, JL, et al. (1991a). A comparison of breastfeeding data from the National Surveys of Family Growth and the Ross Laboratories Mothers' Surveys. *Am J Public Health*, 81:1049-52.

Ryan, AS, Rush, D, Krieger, FW, Lewandowski, GE (1991b). Recent declines in breast-feeding in the United States, 1984 through 1989. *Pediatrics*, 88(4):719-27.

Saarinen, UM (1982). Prolonged breastfeeding as prophylaxis for recurrent otitis media. *Acta Paediatr Scand*, 71:567-71.

Salih, MA, el Bushra, HM, Satti, SA, Ahmed, M el-F, Kamil, IA (1993). Attitudes and practices of breastfeeding in Sudanese urban and rural communities. *Trop Geogr Med*, 45(4):171-74.

Sears, WM (1986). *Becoming a Father*. La Leche League International: Franklin Park, IL.

Sears, WM, Sears, M (1993). *The Baby Book*. Little, Brown: Boston.

Selby, M (1977). Fostering breastfeeding: A pediatric program. *Keeping Abreast J*, July-September:180-85.

Singhania, RU, Kabra, SK, Bansal, A (1990). Infant feeding practices in educated mothers from upper socio-economic status. *Indian J Pediatr*, 57(6):591-93.

Snell, BJ, Krantz, M, Keeton, R, Delgado, K, Peckham, C (1992). The association of formula samples given at hospital discharge with the early duration of breastfeeding. *J Hum Lact*, 8(2):67-72.

Starbird, EH (1991). Comparison of influences on breastfeeding initation of firstborn children, 1960-69 vs. 1970-79. *Soc Sci Med*, 33:627-34.

Subbulakshmi, G, Udipi, SA, Nirmalamma, N (1990). Feeding of colostrum in urban and rural areas. *Indian J Pediatr*, 57(2):191-96.

Takala, AK, Escola, J, Palmgren, J, et al. (1989). Risk factors of invasive Haemophilus influenzae type b disease among children in Finland. *J Pediatr*, 115:694-701.

Teele, DW, Klein, JO, Rosner, B (1989). Epidemiology of otitis media during the first seven years of life in children in greater Boston: A prospective, cohort study. *J Infect Dis*, 160:83-93.

Tuttle, CR, Dewey, KG (1994). Determinants of infant feeding choices among Southeast Asian immigrants in northern California. *J Am Diet Assoc*, 94(3):282-86.

United Nations Children's Fund (UNICEF) (1992). *Hospital Self-Appraisal Tool for the WHO/UNICEF Baby-Friendly Hospital Initiative*. United Nations: New York.

U.S. Department of Agriculture, Food and Nutrition Service (1988). *Promoting breastfeeding in WIC: A compendium of practical approaches*. U.S. Government Printing Office: Washington, DC.

Vestermark, V, Hogdall, CK, Plenov, G, Birch M (1991). Duration of breastfeeding. *Ugeskr Laeger*, 153(43):3010-12.

Virtanen, S, et al. (1991). Infant feeding in Finnish children <7 years of age with newly diagnosed IDDM. *Diabetes Care*, 14:415-17.

Wade, C (1994). Lecture, Emory University Conference, Atlanta.

Walker, M (1992). Why aren't more mothers breastfeeding? *Childbirth Instr*, Winter.

The Washington Post (1981). Breastfeeding ruled a constitutional right, July 18.

Weile, B, Rubin, DH, Krasilnikoff, PA, Kuo, HS, Jekel, JF (1990). Infant feeding patterns during the first year of life in Denmark: Factors associated with the discontinuation of breast-feeding. *Clinical Epidemiol*, 43(12):1305-11.

Williams, EL, Pan, E (1994). Breastfeeding initation among a low income multiethnic population in northern California: An exploratory study. *J Hum Lact*, 10(4):245-51.

Williamson, NE (1990). Breastfeeding trends and the breastfeeding promotion program in the Philippines. *Int J Gynaecol Obstet*, 31 (Suppl 1):35-41; discussions, 43-45.

World Alliance for Breastfeeding Action (WABA) (1993*). The Mother-Friendly Workplace Initiative Action Folder*. Pernang, Malaysia.

World Health Organization (WHO) (1981*). Resolution of the 34th World Health Assembly International Code of Marketing of Breast-milk Substitutes*, Geneva: Fifteenth Plenary Meeting.

WHO (1989). *Promoting and Supporting Breastfeeding: The Special Role of Maternity Services*, Geneva.

World Summit for Children (1990). *Innocenti Declaration*. Florence, Italy.

Wright, AL, Holberg, CJ, Martinez, FD, et al. (1989). Breastfeeding and lower respiratory tract illness in the first year of life. *Br Med J*, 244:946-50.

Wright, AL, Holberg, CJ, Taussig, LM, et al. (1988). Infant feeding practices among middle-class Anglos and Hispanics. *Pediatrics*, 82:496.

ADDITIONAL READINGS

Andrew, EM, Clancy, KL, Katz, MG (1980). Infant feeding practices of families belonging to a prepaid group practice health-care plan. *Pediatrics*, 65(5):978-88.

Arkin, EB, Cooper, L, Jordan, L (1987). Healthy Mothers, Healthy Babies Coalition. *Public Health Currents*, 27(2).

Auerbach, KG, Pessyl, MM (1992). A baby-friendly environment: More than a dream? *J Hum Lact*, 8(4):189-92.

Bagwell, JE, Kendrick, OW, Stitt, KR, Leeper, JD (1993). Knowledge and attitudes toward breastfeeding: Differences among dietitians, nurses, and physicians working with WIC clients. *J Am Diet Assoc* 93:801-4.

Baldwin, E (1993). Is breastfeeding really a visitation issue? *Mothering*, Fall:84-87.

Baranowski, T, Rassin, D, Richardson, J, Bee, D, Palmer, J (1990). Expectancies of infant feeding methods among mothers in three ethnic groups, *Psychol Health*, 1-17.

Beasley, A (1991). Breastfeeding studies: Culture, biomedicine, and methodology. *J Hum Lact*, 7(1):7-14.

Berger, A, Winter, ST (1980). Attitudes and knowledge of secondary school girls concerning breast feeding. *Clinical Pediatr*, 19(12):825-26.

Berkowitz, EN, Kerrin, RA, Hartley, SW, Rudelius, W (1994). *Marketing*. Irwin: Boston.

Boehl, D (1992). *Breastfeeding Does Make a Difference*: No. 64, La Leche League International: Franklin Park, IL.

Breastfeeding and weaning in Mexico and the U.S. (1986). *Nutr Rev*, 44(3):104-6.

Brown, F, Lieberman, J, Winston, J, Pleshette, N (1960). Studies in choice of infant feeding by primiparas. *J Am Psychosomatic Soc*, 22(6):421-29.

Dillman, DA (1978). *Mail and Telephone Surveys: The Total Design Methods*. Wiley: New York.

Gibson, VM (1993). Employer support for nursing mothers yields numerous benefits. *HR Focus*, 17.

Gielen, AC, Faden, RR, Paige, DM, Buxton, KE, Brown, CH, Chwalow, AJ (1988). Breastfeeding promotion in obstetrical care practices: Limitations and opportunities. *Patient Educ Couns*, 12:5-12.

Giugliani, ERJ, Issler, RMS, Justo, EB, Seffrin, CF, Hartmann, RM, Carvalho, NM (1992). Risk factors for early termination of breastfeeding in Brazil. *Acta Paediatr*, 81:484-87.

Gotsch, G (1989). La Leche League—Can breastfeeding become the cultural norm? *Baby Talk*, 48, 50.

Greenbank, GE, Hafez, S (1979). Factors influencing breastfeeding. *J Nurs Care*, 6-9.

Greer, C (1991). An explanation of the WIC program. *Ashville Citizen-Times*: 1C-2C.

Gussler, JD, Briesemeister, LH (1980). The insufficient milk syndrome: A biocultural explanation. *Med Anthropol*, 4:145-74.

Hanson, A, Bergstrom, S (1990). The link between infant mortality and birth rates: The importance of breastfeeding as a common factor. *Acta Paediatr Scand*, 79:481-89.

Heffern, D (1990). Reminders for building confidence in breastfeeding moms. *MCN*, 15:267.

Hill, PD, Aldag, JC (1993). Insufficient milk supply among black and white breastfeeding mothers. *Res Nurs Health*, 16(3):22-23.

Houston, MJ, Howie, PW (1981). Home support for the breastfeeding mother. *J Health Visitor*, 54(6):378.

Humenick, SS (1992). A call for the lactation initiator: Setting the standard. *J Hum Lact*, 8(3):121.

Jackson, DA, Imong, SM, Wongsawasdii, L, Silprasert, A, Preunglampoo, S, Leelapat, P, Drewett, RF, Amatayakul, K, Baum, JD (1992). Weaning practices and breastfeeding duration in northern Thailand. *Br J Nutr*, 67(2):149-64.

Kistin, N, et al. (1990). Breastfeeding rates among black urban low-income women: Effect of prenatal education. *Pediatrics*, 86:741-46.

Klaus, M, Kennell, JH (1982). *Parent–Infant Bonding*. Mosby: St Louis.

Kurinij, N, et al. (1979). Does maternal employment affect breastfeeding? *Am J Pub Health*, 19:1247-50.

La Leche League International (1990). *What Is La Leche League?* No. 3. LLLI: Franklin Park, IL.

Lazarov, MS, Fleshood, L, et al. (1989). Innovative approches to the promotion of breastfeeding. *J Tenn Med Assoc*, 9:486.

Levinson, JC (1990). *Guerrilla Marketing Weapons*. Penguin: New York.

Libbus, MK (1992). Perspectives of common breastfeeding situations: A known group comparison. *J Hum Lact*, 8(4):199-203.

Martinez, GA (1983). 1981 milk feeding patterns in the United States during the first 1 to 3 months of life. *Pediatrics*, 71(2):166-70.

Martinez, GA (1984). 1984 milk feeding patterns in the United States. *Pediatrics*, 76:1004-8.

Martinez, GA, Nalezienski, JP (1979). The recent trend in breast-feeding. *Pediatrics*, 64(5):686-92.

McClurg-Hitt, D, Olsen, J (1994). Infant feeding decisions in the Missouri WIC program, *J Hum Lact*, 10(4):253-56.

Millard, AV (1990). The place of the clock in pediatric advice: Rationales, cultural themes and impediments to breastfeeding. *Soc Sci Med*, 31:211-21.

Minchin, M (1989). *Breastfeeding Matters*. George Allen and Urwin: N. Sydney, Australia.

Morse, JM (1990). Euch, Those are for your husband! Examination of cultural values and assumptions associated with breastfeeding. *Health Care Women Int*, 11:223-32.

Nadel, EL (1993). Breastfeeding promotion in an urban New Jersey WIC office. *J Hum Lact*, 9(2):140-42.

Naggan, L, Forman, MR, Sarov, B, Lewando-Hundt, G, Zangwill, L, Chang, D, Berendes, HW (1991). The Bedouin Infant Feeding Study: Study design and factors influencing the duration of breastfeeding. *Paediatr Perinat Epidemiol*, 5(4):428-44.

Peterson, CE, DaVanzo, J (1992). Why are teenagers in the United States less likely to breast-feed than older women? *Demography*, 29(3):431-50.

Ryckman, LL (1991). If breast is best for baby, why does the bottle prevail? *Ashville Citizen-Times*:1C-2C.

Serdula, M, et al. (1991). Correlates of breastfeeding in low-income populations of whites, blacks and Southeast Asians. *J Am Diet Assoc*, 91:41-45.

Shoham-Yakubovich, I, Pliskin, JS, Carr, D (1990). Infant feeding practices: An evaluation of the impact of a health education course. *Am J Public Health*, 80(6):732-34.

Sugarman, M (1989). Cultural attitudes that interfere with breastfeeding choices. *Breastfeeding Abstracts*, 8(40):19-20.

Terek, M (1992). WIC News. *Medela Rental Roundup*. Medela: McHenry, IL.

U.S. Department of Health and Human Services, Public Health Service (1990). *Promoting Health/Preventing Disease: Objectives for the Nation*. U.S. Government Printing Office: Washington, DC.

Van Esterick, P (1989). *Beyond the Breast–Bottle Controversy*. Rutgers University Press: New Brunswick, NJ.

Victora, CG, Tomasi, E, Olinto, MT, Barros, FC (1993). Use of pacifiers and breastfeeding duration. *Lancet*, 341 (BB42):404-6.

CHAPTER 2

Advantages of Breastfeeding and Hazards of Artificial Feeding

SECTION A

Advantages of Breastfeeding

Rebecca F. Black, MS, RD/LD, IBCLC
Jill L. Goode, RD/LD

LEARNING OBJECTIVES

At the completion of this section, the learner will be able to do the following:

1. Discuss four infant benefits from breastfeeding.
2. Discuss two maternal benefits from breastfeeding.
3. Discuss three benefits to society from breastfeeding.

OUTLINE

I. Benefits to the Child

   A. Nutritional benefits of human milk

      1. Species specificity

      2. Lower renal solute load of human milk

      3. Nutrient bioavailability

      4. Optimal caloric utilization

   B. Nonnutritive benefits of human milk

      1. Colonization of digestive system

      2. Defenses in human milk

      3. Anti-inflammatory agents

      4. Reduction in infections

   C. Developmental benefits of human milk

      1. Development of gastrointestinal tract

      2. Development of visual acuity

3. Enhancement of cognitive development
4. Development of the jaw
5. Benefits as a result of mode of feeding
6. Potential for reduced child abuse and neglect
7. Adaptability to changing needs

II. Benefits of Breastfeeding for Parents

A. Convenience
B. Cost
C. Hormonal elevations
D. Natural means of contraception
E. Reduction in chance of maternal cancer
F. Reduction in maternal weight

III. Benefits to Society and the Global Community

A. Decrease in infant morbidity and mortality
B. Reduction of health-care costs
C. Save natural resources
D. Reduction in world hunger
E. Ecological implications

PRE-TEST

For questions 1 to 5, choose the best answer.

1. The long-chain fatty acids and cholesterol in breastmilk
   A. cause infants to have hyperlipidemia as adults.
   B. aid in the myelinization of nervous tissue.
   C. are difficult for infants to digest.
   D. support rapid musculoskeletal growth.

2. Breastmilk composition
   A. remains the same throughout the lactational period.
   B. decreases in nutrient content as the infant's gastrointestinal system adapts to digest and absorb nutrients.
   C. lacks the antibodies needed to fight infection.
   D. adapts to the changing needs of the infant.

3. The production of formula results in
   A. a decrease in landfill space.
   B. an increase in woodland areas.
   C. less use of tin plate.
   D. more natural resource availability.

4. _____ is a nonpathogenic bacteria that colonizes in the digestive system and reduces the growth of other bacteria.
   A. Lactoferrin
   B. Salmonella
   C. E. coli
   D. Lactobacillus

5. The protein content of breastmilk
   A. increases renal solute load.
   B. is in excess of the amounts the infant needs.
   C. is completely utilized by the infant.
   D. does not meet the needs of newborns and, therefore, must be supplemented.

For questions 6 to 10, choose the best answer from the following key:

    A. Docosahexanoic acid (DHA)   **D. Oxytocin**
    B. Lactobacillus   **E. Prolactin**
    C. Inositol

6. Enhances the synthesis and secretion of surfactant in immature lung tissue.

7. A hormone that promotes feelings of closeness and mothering behavior.

8. Reduces the growth of E. coli, salmonella, and shigella.

9. Needed for growth and development of the brain.

10. Acts as a natural tranquilizer.

For questions 11 to 16, choose the best answer.

11. The hormonal elevation of prolactin during breastfeeding
    A. causes mothers to be alienated from their infant.
    B. excites the mother and helps her cope with the stress of caring for a newborn.
    C. promotes feelings of closeness and mothering behavior.
    D. increases the duration of the menstrual cycle.

12. Breastfed infants often
    A. need more diapers because of increased waste excretion.
    B. cry more because of increased contact with the mother.
    C. cry less because of lack of physical contact.
    D. need fewer diapers because of less waste excretion.

13. Breastfed infants have a/an
    A. increased risk of infection.
    B. high levels of antibodies.
    C. decreased response to vaccines.
    D. array of defenses that aid in the colonization of common microbial pathogens.

14. Live cells include
    A. lymphocytes.
    B. polymorphonucleocytes.
    C. macrophages.
    D. none of the above.
    E. all of the above.

15. This anti-infective agent is thermal and acid stable and acts as a noninflammatogenic.
    A. Macrophages
    B. Polymorphonucleocytes
    C. Secretory IgA
    D. Lactoferrin

16. This component of breastmilk comprises 90% of cellular components, secretes lysozyme and growth factors, and participates in bacteria phagocytosis.
    A. Polymorphonucleocytes
    B. Lymphocytes
    C. Lactoferrin
    D. Macrophages

For questions 17 to 20, choose the best answer from the following key:
    A. if responses 1, 2, and 3 are correct   **D. if response 4 is correct**
    B. if responses 1 and 3 are correct   **E. if all are correct**
    C. if responses 2 and 4 are correct

17. Benefits breastfeeding provides to the society and the global community are
    1. reduction in health-care costs.
    2. reduction in world hunger.
    3. reduction in infant morbidity and mortality.
    4. reduction in natural resources.

18. Breastmilk contains
    1. antimicrobial agents.
    2. immunological agents.
    3. anti-inflammatory agents.
    4. malignant neoplastic agents.

19. Human milk is designed
    1. to be species specific.
    2. to support rapid musculoskeletal growth.
    3. to support growth and development of the central nervous system.
    4. to meet the specific needs of all mammalian species.

20. Breastfeeding benefits parents in that it
    1. generally protects against pregnancy during the first six months postpartum.
    2. reduces the risk of breast cancer.
    3. costs less than formula.
    4. is convenient and always available without the need for preparation.

Benefits to the Child

Human milk is a nutritional, immunological, and developmental fluid. The benefits of breastfeeding to the infant, mother, family, and society are numerous and impressive. Martha Brower, registered dietitian and lactation consultant, summarizes breastfeeding's qualities in the following statement:

BREASTFEEDING: A PROACTIVE APPROACH TO HUNGER

Breastfeeding is a very potent and underutilized weapon against hunger and malnourishment in babies and young children. Human milk provides a unique blend of nutrients, nurturing delivery system, immunity factors, and cost-free supply that is self-replenishing. It is a priceless commodity that transcends the barriers of poverty, social class, disease, and homelessness. Even malnourished mothers produce milk of excellent quality, unequaled by even the best artificial commercial formula.

Breastfeeding requires only that a mother and baby are able to be together. It does not require refrigeration, storage facilities, good sanitation, supplies, can openers, or electricity. (As the mother who was trapped in a cave in the Rocky Mountains during a blizzard with her infant can testify—although she had NO food or water for several days, she was able to successfully feed her baby, who was in perfect health when they were found.) Breastfeeding frees parents from worry about limited purchasing power (depriving others in the family if the baby is adequately fed), the need for an address (for WIC deliveries), poor access to medical care (breastfed babies are much healthier, even when living in the worst of conditions), and unnecessary illness (babies are protected by their mothers' immune systems as well as their own developing systems).

Breastfeeding suppresses a mother's fertility. Although in this country health-care providers are reluctant to acknowledge this effect, it is real and readily recognized as a free family planning aid in other countries. ANY reduction in the fertility of impoverished women, who struggle daily just to meet the needs of their families, will help stretch resources available to them.

Finally, the superior brain architecture resulting from natural feeding provides impoverished children with the cognitive ability to transcend the barriers of poverty. For mothers to succeed in breastfeeding their babies, the following must happen:

- Mothers must first value breastfeeding—many currently believe that it does not matter.
- Mothers need to receive timely support and knowledgeable assistance to fully implement a breastfeeding decision.
- Mothers need protection from half-truths, harmful advice, and misinformation that can interfere with successful attainment of breastfeeding goals.

Breastfeeding is a proactive approach to hunger management. Mothers develop a pride in their ability to provide for their infants in a way that money cannot buy. Often, this seed of accomplishment matures in unexpected but gratifying ways. The 1984 Surgeon General's Report, the Year 2000 Goals, and the Innocenti Declaration (signed by the U.S. representative) all contain increased breastfeeding initiation and duration rates as goals. Preventive health care begins with breastfeeding. The brains built today will make the world of tomorrow. Human milk has stood the test of time.

Source: Martha Grodrian Brower, RD, IBCLC (Kettering, OH).

NUTRITIONAL BENEFITS OF HUMAN MILK

Species Specificity

As with all mammalian species, human milk provides a unique blend of nutrients that are specific for the human species (see Table 2A–1). It contains an abundance of compounds including sugars, trace elements, electrolytes, simple and complex proteins, glycoproteins and peptides, vitamins, lipids, nucleotides, and living cells (macrophage, lymphocytes, neutrophils, etc.) (Albertson, 1989). Formula companies, scientists, researchers, and others lack the ability to exactly reproduce live cells.

Breastmilk contains:

- Docosahexanoic acid (DHA) needed for growth and development of the brain and retina, myelinization of nervous tissue.
- Cholesterol, which enhances the myelinization of nervous tissue.
- Taurine, the second most abundant amino acid in human milk (Rassin, 1978), functions in bile acid conjugation and may function as an inhibitory neurotransmitter and as a membrane stabilizer.
- Choline (B vitamin), which may enhance memory.
- More than 100 enzymes, such as lipases, that are important in digestion and absorption.
- Citrate, which enhances the absorption of iron.
- Lactoferrin, which sequesters iron so that the iron is unavailable for bacterial growth.
- Inositol, a component of membrane phospholipids, which enhances the synthesis and secretion of surfactant in immature lung tissue.
- Polysaccharides and oligosaccharides, which inhibit bacterial binding to mucosal surfaces.
- Proteins, such as α-lactalbumin, which supply amino acids to the infant, sythesize lactose in the mammary gland, and bind calcium and zinc.

The mammary gland is surrounded by lymph nodes and plasma from which needed nutritive (vitamins and minerals as well as macronutrients) and immune components for maternal milk can be obtained. The mammary gland can also synthesize fatty acids, proteins, and carbohydrates.

Mammalian milk is designed to meet distinctive nutritional needs for growth and development of each specific species (Bocar, 1993):

Table 2A–1 Nutrients in Human Milk with Specific Functions in the Newborn

Nutrient	Function
Long-chain polyunsaturated fatty acids	Brain development, membrane structure and function
Carnitine	Oxidation of fatty acids in mitochondria
Taurine	Bile acid conjugation, needed for brain development, functions as a membrane stabilizer
Polysaccharides, oligosaccharides	Inhibit bacterial binding to mucosal surfaces

- Bovine (cow's) milk supports rapid musculoskeletal growth.
- Human milk supports growth and development of the central nervous system and brain. See Module 3, *The Science of Breastfeeding*, Chapter 2, for more information.

Lower Renal Solute Load of Human Milk

Renal solute load is defined as the sum of solutes that must by excreted by the kidney. It consists of nonmetabolizable dietary components (such as electrolytes), ingested in excess of body needs and metabolic end products (mainly nitrogenous compounds from protein digestion and metabolism). The solute concentration of a feeding is of little value in predicting its renal solute load.

The potential renal solute load (PRSL) of infant feedings has been related to the incidence of hypernatremic dehydration, which was highest when evaporated milk formulas were commonly used. Hypernatremic dehydration as a cause of diarrhea and dehydration resulting in hospitalization declined dramatically as formulas with lower PRSL were used (Finberg, 1989).

The PSRL refers to dietary-origin solutes that would need to be excreted if none were diverted into new tissue synthesis and none lost through nonrenal routes. The PSRL can be calculated by adding the dietary intakes of sodium, chloride, potassium, and phosphorus (expressed as mMol—to convert mg to mMol divide sodium by 23, chloride by 35, potassium by 39, and phosphorus by 31) and the dietary protein divided by 175 or nitrogen divided by 28.

$$PRSL = mMol\ Na + mMol\ CL + mMol\ K + mMol\ P + (Nitrogen \div 28)$$

or

$$PRSL = mMol\ Na + mMol\ CL + mMol\ K + mMol\ P + (Protein \div 175)$$

To estimate the renal solute load the following equation is used:

$$RSL\ est = PRSL - (0.9 \times gain\ in\ grams)$$

To account for nonrenal losses and protein and minerals used, for growth, a formula of 0.9 times the grams of weight gained per day is used (Widdowson & Dickerson, 1964).

To complete the picture of the renal solute load, urinary concentration must then be predicted. When all of the above is taken into consideration, the renal solute load for a healthy, 5.5 kg infant consuming 0.82 liter/day of breastmilk and gaining 30 g/day is 49 mOsm/day. For the same infant receiving milk-based formula, the renal solute load is 84 mOsm/day and for evaporated milk formula, 186 mOsm/day.

It is particularly important to consider renal solute load in infant feeding when the following occur: low fluid intake, abnormally high extrarenal water losses (fever, elevated environmental, temperature, hyperventilation, diarrhea), and impaired renal concentrating ability (renal disease, protein-energy malnutrition, diabetes insipidus). Therefore, for healthy infants fed human milk or formulas, renal solute load considerations are rarely important. However, in an infant with a febrile illness, low intake, and no weight gain, negative water balance can occur. Life-threatening water loss would occur more quickly in an evaporated milk-fed infant than a milk-based, formula-fed infant, with the breastfed infant having the best protection from such an occurrence (Fomon, 1993).

Nutrient Bioavailability

Three major factors contribute to the nutritional status of exclusively breastfed infants: (1) nutrient stores, especially those accumulated in utero, (2) nutrient intake (concentration of nutrients, milk volume, and bioavailability of nutrients), and (3) nutrient utilization, which is affected by environmental and genetic factors. The bioavailablilty of nutrients in human milk influences the amount of nutrient absorbed by the infant.

An example of a vitamin with high bioavailability is folate. Fifty percent more folate is needed by infants fed formula rather than breastmilk to maintain an equivalent folate status throughout the first year (Axelsson et al., 1989; Butte et al., 1984; Dewey & Lönnerdal, 1983; Elk & Magnus, 1982).

Minerals with high bioavailability include iron and copper. The daily intake of copper in exclusively breastfed infants ranges from 0.03 to 0.26 mg/day (Salmenpera et al., 1986)—less than the Food and Nutrition Board's estimated safe and adequate daily dietary intake of 0.4 to 0.6 mg/day for infants aged 0 to 6 months (NRC, 1989). Yet, ceruloplasmin and serum copper consistently rose during exclusive breastfeeding for 12 months (Salmenpera et al., 1986). No case reports of copper deficiency in breastfed infants have been reported (IOM, 1991).

Iron levels in mature human milk are estimated to be 0.3 grams/liter ±1 standard deviation, with a range of 0.2 to 0.9 grams/liter (Picciano & Guthrie, 1976; Siimes et al., 1979). Fifty percent of iron from human milk is absorbed compared to 7% and 4% from iron-fortified formula and cereals respectively. Iron is bound to lactoferrin, lipids, and citrate for improved bioavailability (see Table 2A–2).

Optimal Caloric Utilization

Breastfed infants consume fewer kcal/kg body weight than their formula-fed counterparts throughout the first year (Axelsson et al., 1989; Butte et al., 1984; Dewey & Lönnerdal, 1983; Dewey et al., 1991, Shepherd & Walker, 1988). In industrialized countries, they have been reported to gain weight more quickly with a leveling off in weight below formula-fed infants. Growth of exclusively breastfed infants in industrialized countries, plotted on NCHS growth curves (based primar-

Table 2A–2 Enzymes in Human Milk with Nutritional Functions

Enzyme	Function
Amylase	Digestion of polysaccharides
Lipoprotein lipase	Provides lipid constituents of milk
Lipase (bile salt–dependent)	Digestion of fat triacylglycerol
Proteases	Proteolysis
Xanthine oxidase	Iron, molybdenum carrier
Glutathione peroxidase	Selenium carrier and anti-oxidant
Alkaline phosphatase	Zinc, magnesium carrier
Anti-proteases	Protection of bioactive components (growth factors, hormones, enzymes, immunoglobulins)
Sulfhydryloxidase	Maintains structure and function of milk proteins

Source: Adapted from Institute of Medicine (1991) and Hamosh (1989).

ily on formula-fed infants) show declines in the third to fourth month postpartum (Chandra, 1982; Czajka-Narins & Jung, 1986; Dewey et al., 1990; Duncan et al., 1984; Forsum & Sadurskis, 1986; Garza et al., 1987b; Hitchcock et al., 1985; Saarinen & Siimes, 1979; Salmenpera et al., 1985; Whitehead & Paul, 1984). But when size at birth is controlled, differences in linear growth are small (Czajka-Narins & Jung, 1986; Dewey et al., 1989; Hitchcock & Coy, 1989; Nelson et al., 1989), with weight for length lower for breastfed than formula-fed infants after six months (Czajka-Narins & Jung, 1986; Dewey et al., 1989; Hitchcock & Coy, 1989). Differences in weight-gain patterns may represent adiposity differences (IOM, 1991).

The significance of the differences in growth seen between human milk-fed and formula-fed infants is not known. Many clinicians believe growth charts based on breastmilk-fed infants are needed. Others argue other biochemical markers, such as amino acid profiles, may be more important as researchers seek to understand the significance of formula and human milk nutrient concentrations' effect on growth and development. For more information on nutrient intake and growth of human milk-fed infants, see Module 3, *The Science of Breastfeeding*, Chapter 2.

NONNUTRITIVE BENEFITS OF HUMAN MILK

Nonnutritive substances in human milk include antimicrobial and anti-inflammatory agents, hormones, growth factors, and immunomodulating agents (see Table 2A–3).

Colonization of Digestive System

Breastmilk offers the infant an array of defenses that prevent colonization and proliferation of harmful pathogens and that act as anti-inflammatory agents (Goldman et al., 1991). Polysaccharides and oligosaccharides present in breastmilk inhibit the binding of antigens to mucosal surfaces. This is helpful to a neonate who must transition from an intrauterine life to an extrauterine life and the subsequent gastrointestinal tract exposure to pathogens.

Breastmilk aids in the colonization of the colon with nonpathogenic bacteria. Breastmilk enhances *Bifido bacterium*, a nonpathogenic bacteria, that colonizes in the digestive system. Bifido bacterium reduces the growth of *Escherichia coli*, *Salmonella*, and *Shigella* by producing large quantities of lactic and acetic acid that maintain the pH of the gut at around 5.0. This prevents pathogen-associated bacteria from overgrowing the gut flora (Duffy et al., 1992). Breastmilk also enhances immunological development of the gastrointestinal tract by delivering significant

Table 2A–3   Nonnutritive Substances
in Human Milk

- Live cells
- Anti-infective agents
- Anti-inflammatory agents
- Hormones
- Growth factors
- Other bioactive substances

quantities of living cells (see Table 2A–4) that are believed to play an important role in the gut of the breastfed child (Prentice et al., 1989).

Defenses in Human Milk

Immunologic Agents

Breastmilk contains polymorphonucleocytes, immunoglobulins (IgA, IgG, IgM), T cells, macrophages, and lymphocytes.

Macrophages are found in mucosal areas throughout the mucosal immune system. They are concentrated in the lamina propria just below the epithelium of the mucosa. A high percentage of lamina propria macophages have surface markers, such as class II MHC, which are associated with phagocytic cell activity (Leyva-Cobian & Clemente, 1984). Macrophages are activated by T lymphocytes and are attracted to sites of inflammation by chemotactic factors, thus playing a role in resolving acute inflammation. The macrophage is an active secretory cell having the ability to produce about 100 different substances affecting the inflammatory response (including lactoferin, lysozyme, and complement—mainly C3). Macrophages are phagocytic cells. They can ingest particulate material (phagocytosis) or ingest soluble material (pincytosis), forming pinocytic vesicles for recycling materials. They also serve as regulatory cells. Macrophages in human milk are believed to be involved in the recognition of foreign materials and in the delivery of IgA and lysozyme to critical areas, in the resolution of inflammation, bacterial phagocytosis, and the synthesis and secretion of growth factors.

Lymphocytes comprise 5% to 10% of the cells delivered via breastmilk to the infant. T cells (thymic-derived) make up 59% of the 5% to 10% and transfer systemic immunity from the mother to the infant suggesting that these cells gain entry to the newborn circulation. T cells recognize antigens by complexes on the membrane structure (CD3/TcR). The surface CD3/TcR further differentiates to express CD4 or CD8 on the cell surface. CD4 and CD8 are membrane glycoproteins that bind to class I (CD8) and class II (CD4) major histocompatibility complex (MHC) antigens. The antigen-processing cells internalize and degrade the

Table 2A–4   Living Cells in Human Milk

Macrophages—90% of cellular components
    Secretion of lysozyme
    Bacteria phagocytosis
    Synthesis and secretion of growth factors
    Delivery of sIgA to critical areas

Lymphocytes—5–10% of cellular components
    T cells—59% of the 5–10%
      • Transfer systemic immunity from mother to baby via breastmilk
    B cells
      • Transfer mother's local gut mucosal immunity to the baby
      • Antigen-specific immunoglobulin synthesis and secretion

Granulocytes—0–5%
    Primary type in human milk are neutrophils (polymorphonucleocytes)
    Main function is mammary tissue related
    Numbers decrease after first day
    Numbers increase with an infection

antigens' proteins and present peptides on their cell surface membrane bound to MHC antigens. This interaction of T cells with antigen-presenting cells and the presence of a co-signal generates an activation signal for the T cell. T cells can then generate lymphokines when stimulated in vitro (Keller et al., 1981; Kohl et al., 1980; Lawton et al., 1979). Thus T cells bind to antigens processed into small peptides and bound to MHC antigens on the cells surface of an antigen-presenting cell (like a macrophage or B cell).

B lymphocytes form from progenitor cells in the bone marrow. In early maturation, they rearrange heavy (H) and light (L) chain genes and then synthesize functional H and L chains so that immunoglobulins can be expressed on the cell surface. B cells then migrate into the blood and peripheral lymphoid tissues. Once the surface immunoglobulin interacts with an antigen and receives signals from T cells, the B cell is activated and matures into a plasma cell that produces and secretes large quantities of immunoglobulins. The main immunoglobulin in human milk is secretory IgA (Goldman & Goldblum, 1989). The cells in the mammary gland that produce sIgA originate from B lymphocytes from the small intestine or respiratory tract. They enter the systemic circulation in response to lactogenic hormones and they are transformed to plasma cells that produce sIgA in the breast (Weisz-Carrington et al., 1978). After exposure to antigen, memory B cells are generated. B cells secrete cytokines, which affect growth and differentiation of B cells and T cells and function as immunoregulators.

Once an exposure to an antigen occurs (including via immunization) the T cell generates memory T cells. Memory T cells result in a rapid response to reexposure to the antigen. Breastfed infants show better serum and secretory responses to peroral and parenteral vaccines (Hahn-Zoric et al., 1990).

Secretory Immune System

The lymph nodes are secondary organs of the immune system. The lymph nodes are round, encapsulated structures that in their resting state range from 1 to 25 mm in diameter but enlarge significantly during infection or malignancy. They are usually located at the junction of major lymphatic tracts. Lymph nodes are the central organs in lymphocyte (B and T cells) circulation and serve to filter out particulate foreign matter and tissue debris. Lymphocytes are one type of cell in the immune system. Lymphocytes continuously recirculate through the lymphatic and vascular channel so that they are in dynamic equilibrium in the blood and tissues. Lymph capillaries are abundant in the breast. Lymph capillaries unite to form large lymphatic vessels. Lymphatics are provided with valves to ensure that the lymphatic flow is away from the tissues. (See Figure 2A–1.)

The lymph drainage of the breast is by way of the axillary nodes, subclavicular nodes, and the internal thoracic nodes. Together these three groups of lymph nodes provide superficial drainage, areola and nipple drainage of the subareolar lymph plexus of sappy, and deep drainage of the glandular tissue of the corpus mammae.

The lymph nodes and spleen respond to antigens introduced into the tissues they drain. The gut, lungs, breast, and external mucous surfaces also have areas known as malt- or mucosa-associated lymphoid tissues, which behave somewhat as a separate circuit for recirculation purposes. They are strategically placed so that the lymph from most parts of the body drains through a series of nodes before reaching the thoraic duct, which empties into the left subclavian vein to allow the lymphocytes to recirculate again via the blood.

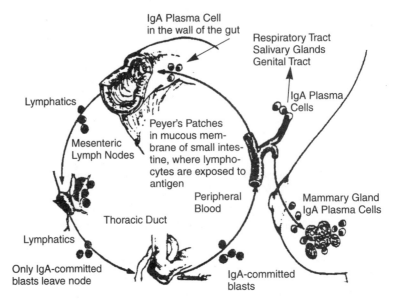

Figure 2A-1   The Secretory Immune System

Precursor B-lymphocytes are exposed to antigens through the specialized epithelium of the Peyer's patches in the lumen of the gut. They are stimulated to divide and migrate into the mesenteric lymph nodes, where they again divide and differentiate into blasts. The IgA-committed lymphoblasts enter the blood stream via the thoracic duct, where further differentiation takes place in contact with T cells. They "home" to sites of secretory antibody production in the gut, in the respiratory tract, and in the late pregnant or lactating mammary gland, where they mature into plasma cells that secrete antibody (IgA). Some of these cells and many macrophages migrate transepithelially into the alveolar lumen.

Source: Reproduced from Roux ME, McWilliams M, Phillips-Quagliate JM: Origin of IgA-secreting plasma cells in the mammary gland. *The Journal of Experimental Medicine,* 1977, 146:1311. Copyright © The Rockefeller University Press. Adapted by Gabbe, S: *Obstetrics—Normal and Problem Pregnancies,* 1991, p. 196. Churchill Livingston: New York. Reprinted with permission.

Maternal responses to antigen exposure over her entire life occurs in the form of immunoglobulin production that passes to the infant via her milk. After delivery, lymphoid tissue in the maternal gut releases IgA precursor cells that "home" to the breast via the mesenteric nodes, thoraic duct, and bloodstream. In the breast, these cells differentiate to specific immunoglobulins which are secreted in her milk. Protection is then provided to the infant at the intestinal level.

The importance of the immune system in breastfeeding and more on how it functions is included in Module 3, *The Science of Breastfeeding,* Chapter 2.

Nonimmunologic Agents

Human milk has a complex system of nonimmunologic, antimicrobial factors that prevent infection:

Nonlactose Carbohydrates—Nitrogen-containing sugars promote the growth of *Lactobacilli bifido bacterium* (Gyllenberg & Roine, 1957; Gyorgy et al., 1974; Smith & Crabb, 1961). Specialized oligosaccharides, such as monosialogangliosides and glucoconjugates, inhibit selected bacterial pathogens from binding to mucosal epithelial cells by serving as receptors (Holmgren et al., 1981; Otnaess et al., 1983). Pneumococous is prevented from attaching to the epithelium of the gastrointestinal tract by oligosaccharides (Goldman et al., 1986).

Lipids—Fatty acids and monoglycerides with antimicrobial properties are effective against enteric pathogens like *Giardia lamblia, E. histolytica, T. vaginalis*, and encapsulated cornaviruses (Resta et al., 1985). The human immunodeficiency virus (HIV-1) has been reported to be destroyed in in vitro experiments by human milk lipids (Orloff et al., 1993).

Protein—Lactoferrin, a whey protein present in human milk throughout lactation, competes with microorganisms for ferric iron (Bullen et al., 1978; Kirkpatrick et al., 1971; Stephens et al., 1980). Lactoferrin is resistant to proteolysis (Brines & Brock, 1983; Samson et al., 1980) and appears to interact with other host-resistant factors in killing or inhibiting bacterial pathogens (IOM, 1991). Lysozyme, another important protein in human milk, also interacts with other host-resistant factors to kill pathogens. Lysozyme is resistant to proteolysis and has been reported to break down bacteria by cleaving peptidoglycans from their cell walls (Chipman & Sharon, 1969). Another protein, which has been reported in human milk, that enhances phagocytosis is fibronectin (Friss et al., 1988).

Anti-Inflammatory Agents

Leukocytes are modified so that inflammatory mediators are not present. There are anti-inflammatory agents in breastmilk that inhibit inflammatory responses in infants (see Table 2A–5). The principle ones are lysozyme, antioxidants (α-tocopherol, cystine, ascorbic acid, alpha-antitrypsin, and catalase) (Goldman et al., 1986), growth factors, enzymes (such as platelet-activating factor [PAF] acetylehydrolase), and cytoprotectives.

Other Cells—Breastmilk contains other cellular environmental agents that infants need, such as hormones, inducers, enzymes, and epidermal growth factors; these reduce the migration of microbes (see Tables 2A–6 and 2A–7). For more specifics on the biochemistry and immunology of human milk, see Module 3, *The Science of Breastfeeding*, Chapter 2.

Reduction in Infections

Because of the large array of defenses that breastmilk offers, breastfed infants have a reduced number of infections and/or less severe infections than formula-fed infants. Reductions are seen in gastroenteritis, diarrhea, respiratory infections, sepsis, otitis media, and urinary tract infections.

Gastroenteritis/Diarrhea

Strong evidence for breastfeedings providing protection against gastroenteritis exists (Howie et al., 1990; Rogan et al., 1987). These benefits may be a result of hygienic factors, specific immune factors (IgA), differences in bacterial flora (Duffy et al., 1986b), nonspecific host factors (lactoferrin, epithelial receptor analogues) (Hanson et al., 1985) and/or the presence of milk mucins (Patton, 1994). The digestive system is colonized with nonpathogenic bacteria *Bifido bacterium lactobacillus*, which reduces growth of *E. coli, Salmonella,* and *Shigella* and is responsible for the characteristic smell of breastfed infants' stools.

Theoretical calculations from a comprehensive worldwide review of morbidity–mortality studies suggest that promoting breastfeeding can reduce diarrheal mor-

Table 2A–5   Anti-Infective Agents

Secretory IgA
- Principal immunoglobulin in breastmilk
- Specific activity against microorganisms and infectious agents (bacterial enterotoxins and rotaviruses)
- Resistant to proteolytic enzymes because of "J" piece (dimer form)
- Stable at low pH

Lactoferrin
- Increases as lactation proceeds
- Bacteriostatic when unsaturated with iron
- Works against *Staphylococcus aurus, E. coli,* and *C. albicans*

Lysozyme
- Thermal and acid stable
- Works against enterobacterial gram positive and E. coli
- Has 300 times the concentration in human milk vs. bovine milk
- B_{12}-binding protein

Table 2A–6   Hormones and Growth Factors

Growth Hormones	Other Hormones
Insulin	Calcitonin
Relaxin	Parathyroid hormone–related peptide
Growth hormone (GH)	(PTHrP)
Prolactin (PRL)	Erythropoietin (Epo)
Adrenal Gland Hormones	Thyroid-stimulating hormone (TSH)
Cortisol	Thyroid gland hormones (T_3 and T_4)
Corticosteroid-binding proteins	Growth Factors
Gonadal Hormones	Epidermal growth factor (EGF)
Estrogen	Transforming growth factor—alpha
Progesterone	Transforming growth factor—beta
Brain–Gut Hormones	Insulin-like growth factors (IGF)
Gonadotropic-releasing hormone (GnRH)	Nerve growth factor (NGF)
Somatostatin	Colony-stimulating factor
GH-releasing hormone	*Bifido bacterium bifidum* growth factor
Thyroid-releasing hormone (TRH)	

tality by 25% in the first 6 months of life and by 8% to 9% in the first 5 years (Feachem & Koblinsky, 1984). For rotavirus-positive gastroenteritis, the relative risk for exclusively breastfed infants was 0.27. For nonspecific gastroenteritis, the relative risk for infants exclusively breastfed 4 months or more was 0.29. In the infants receiving no breastmilk, there was a fivefold increased risk of moderate to severe illnesses. The attack rate for rotavirus-positive gastroenteritis were similar between infants given any breastmilk compared to infants receiving none (Duffy et al, 1986a). However, the severity of clinical symptoms, such as emesis, diarrhea, febrile seizures, and dehydration, were significantly reduced in breastfed infants (Duffy et al., 1992). In one hospital nursery, infants with rotavirus infections were treated with breastmilk, and symptoms subsided by 2 to 3 days in most cases (Grillner et al., 1985).

Necrotizing enterocolitis (NEC) has been shown to be 6 to 10 times more common in formula-fed infants than infants fed breastmilk exclusively and 3 times more

Table 2A-7   Other Bioactive Substances

Factor	Role
Complement factors (C_3, C_4)	Low levels in milk; permit bacteria or other cells to be destroyed (opsonization)
Milk lipids	Neutralize viruses
Antioxidants: ∂-tocopherol, cysteine, ascorbic acid	Counteract inflammatory activity of the immune system
Anti-staphylococcal factor	Inhibits staphylococcal infection in the blood
Bifidus factor	Promotes growth of *bifido* bacteria in the intestinal flora, limits the growth of disease-producing micro-organisms (enteric pathogens)
Antiviral RNAse	Inhibits viral activity
Interferon	Inhibits viral infection
Catalase, glutathione peroxidase	Destroy peroxides
Antitrypsin, antichymotrypsin	Protease inhibitors
Histaminase	Catabolizes histamine, decreasing inflammation
Prostaglandins E_2, F_2a	Inhibit neutrophil degranulation, noninflammatogenic
Nucleotides	Benefit gut flora; enhance immunity and iron absorption

Source: Adapted from Goldman AS, Thorpe LW, Goldblum RM, Hanson LA. Anti-inflammatory properties of human milk. *Acta Paediatr Scand*, 1986; 75:689-95; and Mata, L. Breast feeding, diarrheal disease, and malnutrition in less developed countries. In: Lifshitz, F (ed.), *Pediatric Nutrition, Infant Feeding: Deficiencies, Decreases*. New York: Marcel Dekker, 1982:355-372. Used with permission.

common in infants fed formula and breastmilk. In infants less than 30 weeks gestational age, NEC is 20 times more common in the formula-fed over the exclusively breastmilk-fed infant (Lucas & Cole, 1990). DeCurtis et al. (1987) have also shown a beneficial effect of breastfeeding compared to formula feeding in the prevention of NEC in the human. Furukawa et al. (1993) have identified the presence of platelet-activating factor-acetylhydrolase in human milk (PAF-AH). PAF-AH is an enzyme that metobolizes platelet-activating factor (one of the most pro-inflammatory agents thus far described) to the biologically inactive lyso PAF. Platelet-activating factor has been implicated in the development of certain inflammatory bowel diseases (Whittle & Esplugues, 1989) and along with endotoxin and tumor neorosis factor-alpha has been suggested to play a role in the development of NEC in the newborn (Caplan et al., 1990).

PAF-AH is not present in bovine milk (Furukawa et al., 1993). PAF-AH in human milk survives at a low pH and is believed to be important in preventing the accumulation of PAF in the small intestine. More research will be needed to determine if this enzyme plays a significant role in preventing NEC (see Table 2A-8).

Otitis Media

Exclusive breastfeeding for four or more months has been shown to protect infants from single and recurrent episodes of otitis media (Duncan et al., 1993); they have one-half the occurrence of otitis media compared to formula-fed infants. The

Table 2A-8 Selected Microbial Causes of Diarrheal Illness—Research Shows that Breastfeeding Has a Protective Effect

Cryptosporidium	Pape et al., 1987
Campylobacter jejuni	Ruiz-Palacios et al., 1986
Rotavirus	Jayashree et al., 1988; Duffy et al., 1992
Shigellosis	Clemens et al., 1986; Ahmed et al., 1992
Giardia lamblia	Gendrel et al., 1989
Salmonella enteritidis	Haddock et al., 1991
Ascaris giardia	Gendrel et al., 1988

risk of otitis media (Rogan et al., 1987) and lower-respiratory illness is doubled by not breastfeeding (Wright et al., 1989).

It is unclear by what mechanisms or combination this difference is seen. Contributors to the lower incidence of otitis media may be secretory IgA, prostaglandin (decrease inflammatory response), or positioning while breastfeeding, which minimizes pooling in the eustachian tube. Previous studies suggest the development of otitis media may be closely associated with nasopharyngeal colonization patterns of nontypeable *Haemophilus influenzae* (Faden et al., 1990; Faden et al., 1991). Harabuchi et al. (1994) followed 68 human milk-fed children from birth to 12 months of age to assess the effect of human milk secretory IgA antibody to P6—an outer-membrane protein of nontypeable *H. influenzae* (a frequent cause of otitis media). They found the frequency of isolation of nontypeable *H. influenzae* was directly related to episodes of otitis media and that the level of human milk anti-P6 secretory IgA antibody was inversely related to frequency of isolation of the organism. The authors suggest the protective effect of human milk against otitis media may be partially the result of inhibition of nasopharyngeal colonization with nontypeable *H. influenzae* by specific secretory IgA antibody (Harabuchi et al., 1994).

Urinary Tract Infections

Pisacane et al. (1992) found the relative risk of a urinary tract infection while being breastfed in the first 6 months to be 0.38 in a study with 128 breastfed and 128 controls (formula fed). The urinary tract has mucosal tissue with the products of the secretory immune system "bathing" the area, which may explain how breastfeeding affords protection at a site removed from the gut.

Respiratory Illness

Bottle-fed infants have been shown to have sixfold the risk of respiratory illness compared with infants breastfed three or more months (Howie et al., 1990). The prophylactic effect of breastfeeding helps fight the respiratory syncytial virus (Cunningham et al., 1991). Smoking and formula-feeding synergistically increase the risk of respiratory disease. Breastfeeding has also been found to be protective for serious *H. influenzae* (Hib) disease (Cochi et al., 1986).

Sepsis

Major protection against bacteremia-meningitis has been reported in industrial countries as well as in developing countries. In Atlanta, Georgia, the adjusted risk for bacteremia-meningitis is twelvefold for formula-fed infants in the first six months (Cochi et al., 1986). In Finland, prolonged breastfeeding was protective against bacteremia-meningitis in children under 5 years with an odds ratio of 0.47 when controlling for daycare, history of previous illness, and presence of siblings (Takala et al., 1989). In Pakistan, the risk of neonatal septicemia is 18 times higher among nonbreastfed than partially breastfed infants.

DEVELOPMENTAL BENEFITS OF HUMAN MILK
Development of Gastrointestinal Tract

Human milk stimulates the functional maturation of the gastrointestinal tract and stimulates the baby's own immune protection (Jensen,1989). Enzymes, hormones, and growth factors are present in human milk in concentrations higher than milk from other species and these play important physiologic and protective roles in gut growth and immunity. In animal models, epidermal and neural growth factors in milk (Menard & Arsenault, 1988) and hormones (Koldovsky et al., 1989) contribute to gastrointestinal maturation. Specifically, nerve growth factor, epidermal growth factor, and transforming growth factor—alpha and beta—stimulate cell growth and differentiation of the gastrointestinal tract. Nucleotides have also been implicated in intestinal development (Uauy et al., 1990). Polyamines, which are involved in cell proliferation and differentiation in many tissues, are found in human milk and are believed to act on the intestinal mucosa as well (Pollack et al., 1992). Many intestinal lipases, including bile salt-stimulated lipase and pancreatic amylase, are not mature in the neonate's gut. Breastmilk contains these enzymes and human milk–fed infants demonstrate lower fecal fat losses than formula-fed infants and more efficient triacylglycerol utilization (Blackberg & Hernell, 1993).

Development of Visual Acuity

Docosahexaneoic acid (22:6 Ω-3) is important for the development of photo receptor cells of the retina. In human infants, early Ω-3 (docosahexaneoic acid) accretion is closely linked to development of visual acuity (Uauy et al., 1990, 1992).

Formulas contain precursors to docosahexaneoic acid (a-linolenic acid 18:3 Ω-3) but do not actually contain the long-chain polyunsaturated fats. In preterm infants fed conventional infant formulas, plasma and membrane phospholipids rapidly became depleted of Ω-6 and Ω-3 long-chain polyunsaturated fatty acids in comparison with breastfed infants (Koletzko et al., 1989; Putnam et al., 1982). An enzyme (Δ6 desaturase) is required to convert precursor fatty acids (linoleic and linolenic) to long-chain polyunsaturated fatty acids. Whether this enzyme system is mature in the preterm infant is not known.

In one study of the role of feeding in visual development, both preterm and full-term infants without eye disorders, neurological disorders, or meaningful neonatal morbidity were tested at 57 weeks and at 36 months. The human milk-fed group had better acuity at 57 weeks with the differences most notable for the preterm infants. The formula-fed group had markedly lower stereo acuity and better matching skills than their breastfed counterparts at 36 months. Blood tests correlated improved visual scores at 57 weeks and 36 months with a dietary sufficiency of the Ω-3 long-chain polyunsaturated fatty acids (Birch et al., 1993).

Enhancement of Cognitive Development

Nutrients in human milk support optimal human growth by development of the central nervous system. Myelanization of nervous tissue is enhanced by long-chain fatty acids (docosahexaneoic, Ω-3, and arachidonic, Ω-6) and cholesterol, optimal proportion of amino acids, and optimal levels of vitamins and minerals.

The cognitive development of the infant is complex and influenced by genetic and environmental factors that interact. The educational and socioeconomic characteristics of the family have been reported to have a direct influence on the child's intellectual development (as has the type of feeding received) and so must be controlled for in studies that look at infant feeding's influence on intellectual development (Barros et al., 1986; Seward & Sercula, 1984; Temboury et al., 1994).

Studies demonstrate a relationship between breastfeeding and increased intelligence. In a cohort of preterm infants fed human milk, one half of a standard deviation higher score on intelligence quotient (IQ) testing was noted for the human milk-fed group (IQ increased 8.3 points over those receiving formula) (Lucas et al., 1992).

Higher Bayley scores at 18 months (Morley et al., 1988) and 1 to 2 years (Morrow-Tlucak et al., 1988; Temboury et al., 1994) have been documented in breastfed groups. Developmental testing at 5 years has also shown breastfed infants to score higher than formula-fed infants (Taylor & Wadsworth, 1984).

Development of the Jaw

When malocclusion was the outcome variable and when interviews with mothers (about whether their children have or had braces or bands, obviously need them, or were told by a dentist they were needed) were the method of obtaining the data, the percent of the sample with malocclusion was 33% if not ever breastfed, 28% if breastfed less than 6 months, and 26% with prolonged breastfeeding (Labbok & Hendershot, 1987).

Benefits as a Result of Mode of Feeding

Feeding at the breast offers the infant many benefits not often found with bottle feeding, including:

- Breastfeeding provides increased human and skin-to-skin contact for the infant.
- The infant controls the length of feeding, thus reducing overfeeding.
- The infant's facial muscles are provided a form of exercise that may improve facial–mandibular development as well as dental and periodontal health.
- Respiration is improved, bradycardia lessened, and thermoregulation enhanced when breastfeeding.

Potential for Reduced Child Abuse and Neglect

Caring for an infant may occasionally stir up unconscious feelings of rage and aggressive impulses (Deutsch, 1945). Breastfeeding has been speculated to reduce the incidence of child abuse and neglect. Buranasin (1991) has reported an effect of management of rooming-in on a progressive reduction of deserted children. In the database of 2,000 Thai infants, separation times in the hospital were reduced from 6.3 ± 3.2 hours to 1.62 ± 0.42 hours after rooming-in was begun routinely. This is an area in need of research to support anecdotal claims of reduced abuse and neglect by breastfeeding mothers. Breastfeeding offers continued emotional nurturing for the toddler as he or she separates from mother and explores the world. Perhaps the parent–child relationships formed when breastfeeding reduce conflict and anger in the family.

Adaptability to Changing Needs

Infant Adaptations

Breastmilk composition adapts to the changing needs of the infant:

- Preterm infants' mothers produce milk higher in protein, sodium, chloride, magnesium, and iron (see Table 2A–9).
- As infants' gastrointestinal systems adapt to digestion and absorption of nutrients, the amount of nutrients in breastmilk increases.
- Diurnal and intrafeeding variations provide appropriate nutrients (proportion of fat varies most dramatically).
- Breastfeeding provides a nurturing environment for trust and autonomy to develop.

Maternal Adaptations

Adaptations occur in the mother that are unique to the lactating couplet. The speed of protein synthesis by the mammary gland is increased as are uptakes of amino acids and concentrations of ribonucleic acid (RNA) in the tissue. Muscles are the main supplier of amino acids and are used to meet energy demands or as substrates for the structural, catalytic, and exporting proteins made by the mam-

Table 2A–9   Composition of Preterm[a] Compared with Term[b] Human Milk

Protein	50% to 100% higher during first 4 to 7 weeks after delivery
Sodium	30% to 150% higher during first 4 to 6 weeks after delivery
Chloride	30% to 80% higher during first 3 to 4 weeks after delivery
Potassium	30% to 80% higher during first 3 to 4 weeks after delivery
Calcium, phosphorus, magnesium	Similar to mature human milk
Copper, zinc, iron	Similar during first 2 months
Lactose	Lower than mature human milk
Medium-chain fatty acids	40% to 80% higher during first 3 months
Polyunsaturated fatty acids	40% to 70% higher in colostrum and transitional milk
Water-soluble vitamins	Similar
Bile salt-stimulated lipase	Equal to mature human milk
Amylase	Equal to mature human milk

[a] Preterm milk secreted by women who deliver between 26 and 36 weeks of pregnancy
[b] Mature-term milk secreted by mothers of full-term infants at 6 weeks postpartum.

mary gland. In weaning, the muscle mass recovers protein in undefined amounts (Villalpando & De Santiago, 1990).

Another example of the adaptation that occurs in the lactating mother is the loss of bone density seen during lactation (even in adequately nourished women who use calcium supplements), which is recorded through and after weaning. Evidence exists for bone-density recovery post-weaning. See Module 3, *The Science of Breastfeeding*, Chapter 2 for a discussion of bone-density changes during lactation.

Benefits of Breastfeeding for Parents

CONVENIENCE

Breastfeeding is convenient; it is always available, at the appropriate temperature, and requires no preparation or clean-up. WIC participants in the Southeast interviewed in focus groups, however, did not regard breastfeeding as convenient because only the mother can feed the baby and thus breastfeeding is perceived to interfere with the freedom of the mother (Bryant & Roy, 1989).

COST

Breastfeeding provides at least a threefold cost savings over formula feeding, more if a hypoallergenic formula has to be used. Money diverted from infant feeding can be used to meet other family needs. The government money saved for purchase of formula would be quite substantial even with the cost of peer support leaders and lactation consultants.

HORMONAL ELEVATIONS

During breastfeeding, prolactin and oxytocin levels are elevated in the mother:

- Prolactin promotes feelings of closeness and mothering behavior.
- Oxytocin acts as a natural tranquilizer, helping the new mother cope with the stress of caring for a newborn.

The hormonal changes of lactation include altered follicle-stimulating hormone (FSH) and luteinizing hormone (LH) levels, producing lactational amenorrhea.

NATURAL MEANS OF CONTRACEPTION

Lactational amenorrhea has been shown to provide good protection against pregnancy during the first six months postpartum, even in well-nourished women who are giving their babies supplemental feedings (Lewis et al., 1991). At the Bellagio, Italy, meeting, an international group of scientists reviewed 11 prospective studies and concluded breastfeeding (where the mother remains amenorrheic and feeding frequency and duration are high) to be 98% protective against pregnancy (Labbok, 1989) (see Table 2A–10 and Figure 2A–3). For more information on the lactational amenorrhea method of birth control, see Module 4, *The Management of Breastfeeding*, Chapter 2.

Table 2A-10   Recommended Breastfeeding Behaviors for Optimal Child Survival and Birth Spacing

In an effort to promote optimal child survival and birth spacing, mothers should be encouraged to:

- Begin breastfeeding as soon as possible after the child is born.
- Breastfeed exclusively until the baby is 4 to 6 months old.
- Breastfeed frequently, whenever the infant is hungry, both day and night.
- Continue to breastfeed even if the mother or the baby become ill.
- Avoid using a bottle, pacifiers (dummies), or other nipples.
- Continue to breastfeed while introducing supplemental or semisolid foods.
- Eat sufficient quantities of a variety of foods.

Source: Labbok, MH (1989). *Breastfeeding and Fertility, Mothers and Children Supplement* (8:1). **American Public Health Association: Washington, DC. Reprinted with permission.**

Figure 2A-3

How to determine if a woman can use breast-feeding as a child-spacing method.

Source: Labbok, MH (1989). *Breastfeeding and Fertility, Mothers and Children Supplement* (8:1). American Public Health Association: Washington, DC. Reprinted with permission.

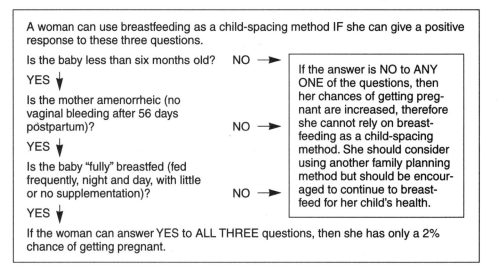

A woman can use breastfeeding as a child-spacing method IF she can give a positive response to these three questions.

Is the baby less than six months old?   NO →

YES ↓

Is the mother amenorrheic (no vaginal bleeding after 56 days postpartum)?   NO →

YES ↓

Is the baby "fully" breastfed (fed frequently, night and day, with little or no supplementation)?   NO →

YES ↓

If the answer is NO to ANY ONE of the questions, then her chances of getting pregnant are increased, therefore she cannot rely on breast-feeding as a child-spacing method. She should consider using another family planning method but should be encouraged to continue to breast-feed for her child's health.

If the woman can answer YES to ALL THREE questions, then she has only a 2% chance of getting pregnant.

REDUCTION IN CHANCE OF MATERNAL CANCER

Protective effects of lactation against breast cancer have been reported. A decreased risk of breast cancer has been found to be associated with an increased number of months of breastfeeding in premenopausal women (Keun-Young et al., 1992). In this study of 521 breast-cancer cases and 521 controls, the relative risk of breast cancer was 0.71 for 1 to 3 months of lactation, dropping to 0.47 for 7 to 9 months. This study did not show an effect for postmenopausal women, which may be because this age group is less likely to have breastfed; thus, there may not have been enough women in the study to show an effect.

Yang et al. (1993) also report no decreased risk for postmenopausal women and a 30% increase in relative risk (1.3) if they never breastfed, a relative risk of 1.0 if they breastfed at least two months, a relative risk of 1.8 if they breastfed only up to one month, and a relative risk of 3.0 if they tried unsuccessfully to lactate. This appears to suggest unsuccessful attempts and duration of less than one month actually increased one's chances of breast cancer.

The largest study to date (5,878 cases, 8,216 controls) by Newcomb (1994) reported the relative risk of premenopausal breast cancer was 0.78 if a woman had lactated. If she first lactated at a maternal age of less than 20, her relative risk of premenopausal breast cancer dropped to 0.54. These authors suggest that if women, who do not breastfeed or do so less than three months, would breastfeed for 4 to 12 months, they could reduce their premenopausal breast-cancer risk by 11%. If lactation occurs for two years (it can be with multiple children), the risk is reduced by 24% (Newcomb, 1994). This study has managed to include large groups of premenopausal women with long durations of breastfeeding. The results suggest that breastfeeding for the first time at a young age (less than 20 years old) and that increased duration (total of 6 months) reduce breast cancer in premenopausal women.

REDUCTION IN MATERNAL WEIGHT

Breastfeeding has long been promoted as a time when weight loss is easier. Maternal recommendations for additional calories for lactation over the nonpregnant, nonlactating state are 500 kcal. Body fat gained during pregnancy is assumed to be mobilized to cover a part of the energy (200 kcal) needed for milk production during a six-month lactation period (WHO, 1985).

Body-composition studies are difficult because of methodological problems; so the energy equivalent of the loss is uncertain, although good evidence that body fat is lost postpartum is available (Butte et al., 1984; Manning-Dalton & Allen; 1983).

Eighty percent of women lost weight while breastfeeding and 20% maintain their weight or gained weight (IOM, 1991; Manning-Dalton & Allen, 1983). The typical weight loss is 0.5 to 1 kg (approximately 1 to 2 pounds) per month in the first 4 to 6 months. Weight loss is not recommended in the immediate postpartum period. Lactating women should weigh themselves after delivery and eat a calorie level that will maintain their weight until the milk supply is well established.

In prolonged lactation, weight loss is enhanced. Dewey et al. (1993) report a loss of 4.4 kg after one year of breastfeeding. Others have found a gradual weight loss of 0.6 to 0.8 kg/month in the first 4 to 6 months of lactation (Butte & Garza, 1986; Butte et al., 1984). Dusdieker, Hemingway, and Stumbo (1994) looked at maternal energy restriction and weight loss in 33 healthy, well-nourished lactating women to determine whether milk production and infant weight gain continues normally over a 10-week interval and whether the macronutrient content of milk (protein and fat) adversely changes. Baseline intake was 2,303 kcalories (kcal) and mean intake during the study was 538 kcal less (1,765 kcal).

Mean daily milk production was reported to be 759 ± 142 ml/day at baseline and 802 ± 187 ml/day at week 10. Infant weight gain averaged 21 g/day or 1.48 ± 0.40 kg overall during the 10-week period. There were no significant differences reported between the percent fat of milk at baseline and at 10 weeks. The mean protein content of the milk at baseline and 10 weeks was similar. The authors conclude that well-nourished, healthy lactating women can safely lose weight at rates of 0.45 kg/week under a program monitored by a health professional skilled at planning a calorically restricted diet that is nutritionally adequate (Dusdieker et al., 1994).

Benefits to Society and the Global Community

DECREASE IN INFANT MORBIDITY AND MORTALITY

Breastfeeding has been shown to decrease infant morbidity and mortality rates, especially in developing countries (Briend et al., 1988; Scott-Emuakpor & Okafor; 1986).

The mortality from bottle feeding in poor nations is at least threefold, even when modern handling of water and sewage is provided (Habicht et al., 1986; Macedo, 1988). Increased risks for diarrheal illness from enteric bacteria and parasites and for respiratory illnesses and lower-respiratory disease when not breastfed have also been shown (Brown et al, 1989; Lanner et al., 1990; Shahid et al., 1988; Tupasi, et al., 1988).

Mortality risks (comparable to Third World countries) from bottle feeding are also higher in poor communities in industrialized nations. Protection against fatal botulism, mortality from diarrhea and respiratory disease and other infections, and protection against sudden infant death syndrome (SIDS) is estimated to account for four infant deaths per 1,000 prevented solely by breastfeeding. Reduced mortality risk from diarrheal and respiratory disease has been shown to be dose-dependent; the higher the number of breastfeedings and the fewer the supplements, the more reduced the mortality (Victoria et al., 1989).

REDUCTION OF HEALTH-CARE COSTS

Breastfeeding has been shown to result in a reduced number of infections in infants, thus reducing the number of hospital stays and doctors' visits. Seventy-seven out of every 1,000 formula-fed infants will be hospitalized during their first four months of life; while only 5 out of every 1,000 breastfed infants will have to be hospitalized (Walker, 1993). Risk of hospitalization has been shown to be greater for respiratory and gastrointestinal illnesses in bottle-fed infants (Chen et al., 1988; Howie et al., 1990).

SAVE NATURAL RESOURCES

Breastmilk is a natural resource, formula is not; and formula requires the use of natural resources in its production. All that breastmilk production requires is approximately 300 to 500 additional calories per day. Harvard economists and physicians estimate that every ounce of human milk to be worth $2.11 (Christopher Wade, MD, lecture at Emory University, 1993).

REDUCTION IN WORLD HUNGER

Many families in developing countries sacrifice family resources to buy formula, thus limiting the amount of food the family has to eat. If the mother breastfeeds the infant, the family is able to purchase more food for the other family members and all are better fed and better nourished. By increasing birth intervals, breastfeeding lowers the world population, thus, enabling limited resources to be shared among fewer people.

ECOLOGICAL IMPLICATIONS

Formula feeding can result in excess use of natural resources and increased waste:

- It takes 200 grams of wood to boil 1 liter of water, so in one year, an artificially fed child would use up at least an extra 73 kgs of wood (Palmer, 1988).
- For every 3 million births of babies who are bottle fed, 70,000 tons of tin plate are used in discarded milk cans (Palmer, 1988). The waste resulting from nipples, bottles and liners, and the paper, glass, and metal waste resulting from packaging and promoting formula decrease landfill space and potentially pollute the environment.
- Lifestyle impact of not breastfeeding: more trips to doctor and pharmacist (time, energy, and money wasted); days off work for one parent if both employed (money wasted).

Breastfeeding can result in a decrease in waste:

- Breastfed babies often need fewer diapers because they excrete less waste during infancy than formula-fed infants.
- Lactating women do not menstruate for longer periods of time and therefore do not require sanitary napkins or tampons (Palmer, 1988).
- Breastfeeding requires only the woman's breast and an infant to be successful so time, energy, and money spent processing artifical feeds are eliminated.

POST-TEST

For questions 1 to 5, choose the best answer.

1. Human milk contains components specific to the human species, including:
    A. casein, lactose, and fatty acids.
    B. docosahexanoic acid, taurine, and inositol.
    C. bile salt-stimulated lipase, lactose, and casein.
    D. bile salt-stimulated lipase, taurine, and lactose.

2. The following determines an infant's nutritional status:
    A. nutrient concentration, bioavailability, and pH.
    B. nutrient concentration, nutrient intake, utilization, and body stores.
    C. nutrient concentration, rate of depletion, weight at birth.
    D. nutrient concentration, weight at birth, pH, and bioavailability.

3. One vitamin with high bioavailability is
    A. calcium.
    B. iron.

   C. folate.

   D. protein.

4. Pick the true statement from the following:

   A. Breastmilk is a more efficient energy source than formula because of its immunologic properties.

   B. Breastmilk is an efficient energy source because of its biochemical composition.

   C. There is no difference in energy intake between exclusively breastfed and formula-fed infants.

   D. Breastfed infants require greater than 120 kcal/kg/day to meet their energy needs.

5. Growth and development may be evaluated by measuring

   A. anthropometrics such as weight, length, and head circumference.

   B. plasma amino and fatty acid levels.

   C. neonatal and infant behavior.

   D. anthropometrics, plasma amino, and fatty acid levels, and behavior and development test results.

For questions 6 to 10, choose the best answer from the following key:

   A. Taurine   **D. Citrate**

   B. Carnitine   **E. Cholesterol**

   C. Polysaccharides

6. Inhibits bacterial binding to mucosal surfaces.

7. Functions as an inhibitory neurotransmitter and membrane stabilizer.

8. Enhances the absorption of iron.

9. Is important in the oxidation of fatty acids in the mitochondria.

10. Found in higher levels in human milk than bovine milk.

For questions 11 to 16, choose the best answer.

11. Enzymes in human milk with nutritional functions include

   A. taurine, carnitine, and amylase.

   B. amylase, lipoprotein lipase, glutathione peroxidase.

   C. cholesterol, casein, and lactoferrin.

   D. lactoferrin, taurine, and lactose.

12. The second most abundant amino acid in human milk, which functions in bile acid conjugation, is

   A. alanine.

   B. carnitine.

   C. glutamine.

   D. taurine.

13. The renal solute load of a feeding is important under the following conditions:

   A. high fluid intake, diarrhea, and fever.

   B. low fluid intake, high extrarenal water losses, impaired renal concentrating ability.

    C. high fluid intake, high extrarenal water losses, impaired renal concentrating ability.

    D. high fluid intake, impaired liver function, high extrarenal concentrating ability.

14. Necrotizing enterocolitis is _____ by _____.

    A. prevented; breastfeeding.

    B. prevented; breastmilk feedings.

    C. minimized; formula feeding.

    D. minimized; breastmilk feedings.

15. T cells and B cells make up 5% to 10% of the cellular components and

    A. secrete lysozyme.

    B. transfer systemic and mucosal immunity from mother to baby via breastmilk.

    C. decrease in number after the first day.

    D. synthesize and secrete growth factors.

16. Breastfed infants show a reduced risk of

    A. otitis media, respiratory illness, and gastrointestinal illness.

    B. contracting yeast infections.

    C. visual acuity development.

    D. enhanced cognitive development.

For questions 17 to 20, choose the best answer from the following key:

    A. if responses 1, 2, and 3 are correct.   **D. if response 4 and correct.**

    B. if responses 1 and 3 are correct.   **E. if all are correct.**

    C. if responses 2 and 4 are correct.

17. Benefits of breastfeeding include

    1. increase in morbidity and mortality.

    2. immunological components that reduce infections.

    3. higher renal solute load than formula or evaporated milk-based feeds.

    4. colonization of the gut with nonpathogenic bacteria.

18. Physical differences in breastfed versus formula-fed infants include:

    1. improved respiration in the breastfeeding infant.

    2. higher antibody response to immunizations.

    3. slower growth by the third to fourth month of age.

    4. longer duration of respiratory synctial virus in the breastfeeding infant.

19. Maternal breast-cancer risk

    1. is reduced in premenopausal women who first lactated before age 20.

    2. is increased in women who breastfed over six months.

    3. is increased in women who never breastfeed.

    4. is reduced in postmenopausal women who formula fed.

20. Benefits of breastfeeding to the global community include:

    1. decrease in infant morbidity and mortality.

    2. reduction of health-care costs.

    3. reduction in world hunger.

    4. a decrease in wastes.

SECTION B

Hazards of Artificial Feeding

Rebecca F. Black, MS, RD/LD, IBCLC
Jill L. Goode, RD/LD

LEARNING OBJECTIVES

At the completion of this section, the learner will be able to do the following:

1. Discuss four hazards of artificial feeding to the infant.
2. Name two infections the infant is at increased risk for contracting if artificially fed.
3. Discuss information that must be provided to parents so an informed decision can be made.

OUTLINE

I. Increased Morbidity and Mortality Rates

    A. Increased risk of infections

        1. Gastrointestinal infections

        2. Upper- and lower-respiratory infections

        3. Botulism

        4. Necrotizing entercolitis

        5. Otitis media

        6. Bacteremia and meningitis

        7. Controversy about the role of breastfeeding in preventing infection

    B. Increased diseases/syndromes

        1. Sudden infant death syndrome

        2. Hypocalcemic tetany

        3. Immune system disorders

4. Chronic liver disease

5. Insulin-dependent diabetes mellitus

6. Allergies

7. Lymphomas

II. Miscellaneous Other Risks of Artificial Feeding

A. Potential for contamination

B. Experimental nature of ingredients

C. Exposure to carcinogens and allergens

D. Risks from type of delivery system

E. Impaired social interaction

F. Impaired cognitive skills

G. Excessive costs

III. Importance of Informed Decision Making

PRE-TEST

For questions 1 to 6, choose the best answer.

1. Caused by the high phosphate loads in formula and causes twitching, convulsions, and atypical seizures.
   A. Hypocalcemic tetany
   B. Sudden infant death syndrome
   C. Chronic liver disease
   D. Elevated renal solute loads

2. Formula-fed infants are less likely than breastfed infants to
   A. be protected against respiratory infection.
   B. develop infant botulism.
   C. become insulin-dependent diabetics.
   D. be hospitalized during their first four months of life.

3. Formula feeding exposes infants to
   A. increased forms of facial muscle exercises.
   B. optimal levels of bioavailable nutrients.
   C. low renal solute loads.
   D. increased risk of contamination.

4. Formula ingredients are regulated through the
   A. Infant Nutritional Support Act of 1970.
   B. Infant Feeding Act of 1970.
   C. Formula Regulatory Act of 1980.
   D. Infant Formula Act of 1980.

5. Formula feeding offers a means for
   A. infants to receive excessive amounts of protein.
   B. poorly educated families to correctly feed their infant.

    C. protection against bacterial contamination.

    D. economically disadvantaged families to inexpensively feed their infant.

6. Formula feeding has been shown to

    A. decrease the intensity of infection in the infant.

    B. lower the incidence of infection in the infant.

    C. prolong the duration of infection in the infant.

    D. solely protect the infant's gastrointestinal tract from infection.

For questions 7 to 10, choose the best answer from the following key:

    A. if responses 1, 2, and 3 are correct.   **D. if only 4 is correct.**

    B. if responses 1 and 3 are correct.   **E. if all are correct.**

    C. if responses 2 and 4 are correct.

7. Which of the following are hazards of formula feeding?

    1. Formula composition alters during shelf life.

    2. Formula feeding may expose infants to carcinogens and allergens.

    3. Formula-fed infants have lower cognitive development.

    4. Formula is composed of living cells and antibodies.

8. Which of the following is a risk of formula feeding?

    1. Increased risk of chronic liver disease.

    2. Increased number of infants with allergies.

    3. Increased likelihood of developing necrotizing enterocolitis.

    4. Increased protection against infection.

9. The experimental nature of formula ingredients results or has resulted in

    1. infants being exposed to a chloride-deficient formula.

    2. a vitamin B deficiency, which causes seizures in some infants.

    3. high amounts of protein, which places infants at risk of hypernatremic dehydration.

    4. infants receiving up to 20 times the amount of iron in breastmilk.

10. Poverty, regardless of whether a nation is considered developed or developing, yields:

    1. increased housing opportunities.

    2. lack of sanitation and potable water.

    3. hygienic conditions.

    4. heavy exposure to microbes.

For question 11 to 16, choose the best answer.

11. Botulism resulting in sudden death

    A. occurs in both breast- and formula-fed infants.

    B. occurs only in formula-fed infants.

    C. occurs in weaning breastfed infants.

    D. occurs in breastfed infants.

12. Formula feeding

    A. increases the risk of necrotizing entercolitis in infants born at less than 30 weeks gestation.

    B. decreases the risk of recurrent otitis media.

    C. decreases the risk of morbidity and mortality.

D. imposes a four- to sixfold lower risk of diarrhea.

E. increases the risk of *H. influenzae* bacteremia.

13. The magnitude of the protective effect in research

    A. is larger in developing countries than in developed countries.

    B. is larger in developed countries than in developing countries.

    C. is smaller in developing countries.

    D. is not different between developed or developing countries.

14. Chance is a potential source of negative results in research because of

    A. the increase in statistical power.

    B. inadequate statistical power.

    C. the increase in sample size.

    D. selection bias.

15. Risk factors for sudden infant death syndrome include:

    A. maternal smoking, prone sleeping position, not breastfeeding.

    B. maternal smoking, not breastfeeding, not drinking.

    C. not drinking, maternal smoking, prone sleeping position.

    D. not breastfeeding, not smoking, not drinking.

16. Formula feeding is associated with

    A. decreased risk of childhood lymphomas.

    B. decreased atopic dermatitis.

    C. increased stooling.

    D. increased risk of insulin-dependent diabetes mellitus.

For questions 17 to 20, choose from the following key:

   A. Hypocalcemic tetany   **C. Baby bottles**

   B. Crohn's and celiac disease   **D. Rotavirus-positive gastroenteritis**

17. Depletion of circulating calcium

18. Formula feeding is a risk factor for developing one of these immune system disorders

19. Formula feeding increases the severity of this illness

20. Can lead to aspiration and dental caries if used incorrectly

Increased Morbidity and Mortality Rates

In the previous section, the material highlighted the many benefits of breastfeeding. In this section, the focus is on the risks of formula feeding or of not breastfeeding. For every 1,000 formula-fed infants, 77 are hospitalized during the first four months of life, while only 5 per 1,000 breastfed infants need to be hospitalized (Cunningham et al., 1991). Morbidity studies show that necrotizing enterocolitis, sepsis, and mortality are reduced when human milk is fed (Eibl et al., 1988; Lucas & Cole, 1990; Uraizee & Gross, 1989). The U.S. National Institute of Environmental Health Sciences estimates an extra 4 per 1,000 will die each year in the United States because they were not breastfed (Rogan, 1989).

Habicht et al. (1986) found the relative mortality risk of not breastfeeding to be 2.67 and 5.20 for households with and without toilets. This translates into 47 and 153 deaths per 1,000 as a result of not breastfeeding. The mortality rate among artificially fed babies has been shown to be 3 to 5 times higher than for breastfed babies (Macedo, 1988). The highest infant mortality in developing countries is in the first months of life (Khan et al., 1993). The major causes of death reported in the early period of life are septicemia and diarrhea. The risk of neonatal septicemia has been reported to be 18 times higher among nonbreastfed than partially breastfed infants (Ashraf et al., 1991). The risk of dying from diarrhea is 23.5 times higher among nonbreastfed compared with exclusively breastfed infants (Victoria et al., 1989).

Hanson and Bergstrom (1990) postulate that infant mortality, birth rates, and breastfeeding are linked. The relationship between decreased child mortality rates and declining birth rates are multifactorial with the evidence suggesting that decreasing infant mortality may lead to decreasing birth rates. They go on to state that breastfeeding leads to decreased infant mortality, increased birth spacing, and decreased fertility. In a viewpoint article, Hanson et al. (1994) reiterate the importance of early exclusive breastfeeding in decreasing infectious disease and death of children and in serving as a strong natural contraceptive, thus increasing the interval between births. They call for campaigns to promote worldwide breastfeeding and they encourage the Catholic Church to promote breastfeeding as a natural contraceptive.

INCREASED RISK OF INFECTIONS

Formula feeding has been shown to increase the incidence, duration, and intensity of infections. Lack of sanitation and potable water, poor housing, unhygienic con-

Figure 2B-1

The cow's perspective on infant feeding.

Source: IBFAN/IOCU (presently known as Consumers International),1990. *Protecting Infant Health—A Health Worker's Guide to the International Code of Marketing of Breast Milk Substitutes*, 6th ed. IBFAN/IOCU: Penang, Malaysia. Reprinted with permission.

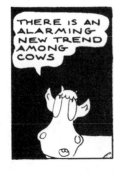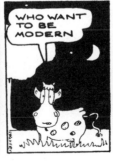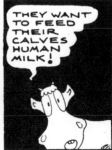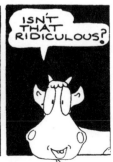

ditions, and excessive exposure to microbes are common where poverty is high. Frequent infections and malnutrition are linked with the deplorable conditions. Infectious diseases are the major cause of high infant mortality in developing countries. Also, the importance of preventing infections to reduce malnutrition is often not recognized. During infections, there is a loss of appetite, loss of nutrients (in diarrhea), and loss of energy (consumed during fever). This added burden may increase the risk of poor growth and/or development (Hanson et al., 1994).

Gastrointestinal Infections

Formula-fed infants have been shown to have a higher rate of gastrointestinal infections. A three- to fivefold increased risk of diarrhea illness exists in formula-fed infants in industrialized nations (Feachem & Koblinsky, 1984). Although breast-feeding will not lower the risk of contact with rotavirus-positive gastroenteritis, it does reduce the severity of the illness (Duffy et al., 1986b). High-iron infant formula tends to promote the development of clinical salmonellosis; however, breast-feeding appears to be protective against salmonellosis (Haddock et al., 1991).

Upper- and Lower-Respiratory Infections

Hospitalization for respiratory infections is more frequent for formula-fed infants (Cunningham et al., 1991). Approximately twice as many formula-fed infants are shown to have episodes of acute chronic bronchitis (de Duran et al., 1991). The risk of death from lower-respiratory tract infections is nearly four times higher in formula-fed infants living in the urban environments of developing nations (Cunningham et al., 1991). Babies who had ever been breastfed had half the hospitalizations for respiratory illness in early childhood than babies formula-fed (Chen et al., 1988). Smoking and bottle feeding act synergistically to raise the risk of serious respiratory illness by three- to fourfold (Chen et al., 1988). Bronchiolitis parainfluenza virus has been found to be higher in infants never breastfed (Welliver et al., 1986) and less severe in infants breastfed at least one month (Porro et al., 1988).

Inositol, a component of membrane phospholipids that enhances the synthesis and secretion of surfactant in immature lung tissue, is present in higher amounts in human milk than in formulas. Preterm colostrum is a rich source of inositol. Inositol significantly reduces the severity of a common occurrence—the preterm infant with respiratory distress syndrome (RDS)—in the neonatal intensive care unit (NICU). Serum inositol levels have been shown to increase with preterm infants fed inositol-rich breastmilk in contrast to formula-fed preterm infants who show no rise in serum inositol levels (Pereira et al., 1990). The lack of inositol in formula places preterm infants consuming it at a higher risk for respiratory failure, bronchopulmonary dysplasia, and retinopathy of prematurity if not supplemented early in life (Hallman et al., 1992).

Botulism

Infant botulism resulting in sudden death occurs only in formula-fed infants. Breastfeeding protects against fatal botulism (Cunningham et al., 1991). A nonfatal botulism has been identified in weaning breastfed infants (Editorial, *Lancet*, 1986; Istre et al., 1986; Spika et al., 1989). This is possibly caused by alterations in gut flora during weaning (Cunningham et al., 1991).

Necrotizing Entercolitis

Infants who are fed formula are 20 times more likely to develop necrotizing entercolitis (NEC) when infants are at least 30 weeks gestational age at birth. For infants born at lower gestational ages, the exclusively formula-fed infants had confirmed NEC 6 to 10 times more often than in those fed breastmilk alone and 3 times more often than those who received formula plus breastmilk (Lucas & Cole, 1990).

Otitis Media

One of the most common illnesses in childhood is otitis media, with 62% of children having at least one episode during their first year of life. Formula feeding increases the risk; however, four months of exclusive breastfeeding decreases the risk of single and recurrent otitis media, and the duration of infections in infants who do contact the illness is decreased as well (Duncan et al., 1993; Fosarelli et al., 1985). Exclusive breastfeeding for more than six months resulted in one third the infection rate in the first three years of life observed in formula-fed infants (Pukander et al., 1985). In 1990, it was reported that 30 million visits to the pediatrician for otitis media occur per year in the United States at a cost of one billion dollars (Facione, 1990).

Bacteremia and Meningitis

Formula feeding imposes an increased risk of *H. influenzae* bacteremia and meningitis for infants living in Finland (Takala et al., 1989). In New York and Connecticut, formula-fed infants had a tenfold risk of hospitalization for bacterial infections and fourfold risk of bacteremia and meningitis.

Several studies in the mid-1980s challenged breastfeeding's role in reducing infections. In a review of 20 epidemiological studies, one group concluded that breastfeeding provides little or no protection in industrialized nations (Bauchner et al., 1986). So strongly is the belief held that breastfeeding is protective for reducing infectious morbidity and mortality in all countries that a debate ensued (Cunningham, 1988, 1989; Leventhal et al., 1986). Cunningham challenged the assertion that no protection was afforded by breastfeeding in industrialized nations (Bauchner et al., 1986) by stating that the authors were biased by selecting articles for review favorable to their hypothesis and that they were more likely to fault the methodology of the article that favored breastfeeding (Cunningham, 1988, 1989).

CONTROVERSY ABOUT THE ROLE OF BREASTFEEDING IN PREVENTING INFECTION

The following is from a 1991 article by Michael Kramer, MD, of McGill University in Montreal:

In developing countries, the epidemiologic evidence that breastfeeding protects against gastrointestinal infection and mortality is overwhelming. Although the mechanisms are less clear, data from developing country settings also indicate protection against morbidity and mortality from respiratory infection. By contrast, the results of studies from modern, industrialized countries have been far less consistent, with several recently published articles failing to find a significant protective effect. These negative results have led to considerable controversy about whether in fact breastfeeding is protective in the latter setting.

What are the reasons for these negative results? One of the most important is probably **effect modification**, i.e., a difference in the magnitude of the protective effect according to setting, not only in developed vs. developing countries, but even within developing or developed countries. Consider the theoretical experiment of raising a group of infants in a germ-free environment. Mode of feeding should have no effect on the incidence of infection in such infants. To the extent that an infant is exposed to potential pathogens, the risk of infection would increase, and so too would the expected benefit of breastfeeding. And in fact, the magnitude of the protective effect has been shown to be considerably larger in developing countries; the protective benefit is much greater in those households where piped water and toilets are not available. A similar phenomenon in developed countries was demonstrated in a recent Arizona study of lower-respiratory-tract infection due to respiratory syncytial virus. In infants of mothers with twelve years or less of education, there were marked differences in infection rate according to the mode of feeding. No such effect was seen among infants of mothers with greater educational attainment.

Chance is another important potential source of negative results, stemming from inadequate statistical power (sample size). When carrying out hypothesis testing (calculating P values), a true protective effect is more likely to be absent in a small sample or, if present, to be statistically nonsignificant. When confidence intervals are recorded, the confidence interval around a point estimate suggesting an impressive protective effect may include the null value; conversely, a point estimate suggesting no benefit, or even a slightly increased risk of infection, could be compatible with an important protective benefit when the sample size is small.

Information bias is a particularly important explanation for negative results. Misclassification of feeding type or the infectious outcome can lead to an association that is biased toward the null. The main problem here is the "lumping" of feeding groups, such as comparing exclusively breastfed infants to all others or combining exclusively breastfed and partially breastfed infants in one group. Another source of information bias toward the null is poor-quality, "noisy" data on feeding and/or infectious outcomes that might stem from inadequate questionnaires or interviews, prolonged maternal recall, or "sloppy" diagnosis of the infectious outcome. A more subtle problem relates to the possible delayed protective effect of breastfeeding. If feeding is classified based on the type given at the time of infection, the non-infected, previously-breastfed infants who are artificially fed at the time of study will be "credited" to the artificial feeding, rather than the prior breastfeeding.

Selection bias can occur because of the way that study subjects are either selected or lost to follow-up. One potential source of selection bias toward the null is selective nonresponse by bottle-feeding mothers whose children develop infection, particularly if those mothers are aware of the study hypothesis and feel guilty when their child develops an infection.

In **confounding bias**, an observed association between feeding type and infection is altered by a third factor that is associated with feeding type and independently affects the risk of infection. Controlling for a covariate that is strongly associated with feeding type but that affects the risk of infection only through infant feeding does not reduce confounding but instead leads to loss of statistical power. For example, control for maternal education, which has no known direct effect on infection (non-confounding correlate), will reduce variation in infant feeding within categories of maternal education and thus could impair the ability to detect a true protective effect of breastfeeding. It would be better to control for those socio-economic aspects of the environment that independently affect the risk of infection, such as crowding, daycare, or other variables more directly linked to exposure to other infected infants and children.

Finally, **publication bias** might also be a source of the recently reported negative results. Although its existence and magnitude cannot be evaluated (because of the absence of data on unsubmitted or unaccepted manuscripts), investigators and editors from developed countries may have been more interested in negative results than positive results, since positive results might have been considered less "newsworthy."

Examination of both negative and positive recent studies from developed countries in the light of these methodologic issues leads to the conclusion that breastfeeding provides measurable protection against infection even in developed country settings. The magnitude of the protective benefit is smaller than in developing countries, however. Future investigators should ensure adequate sample sizes, carefully measure and categorize feeding groups, and avoid "control" for nonconfounding correlates of infant feeding.*

INCREASED DISEASES/SYNDROMES

Sudden Infant Death Syndrome

The cause of sudden infant death syndrome (SIDS) varies, and there are many risk factors. The top three risk factors for SIDS (Mitchell et al., 1991), resulting in 79% of SIDS deaths, are: (1) maternal smoking, (2) prone sleeping position, and (3) not breastfeeding.

It is estimated that one SIDS death per 1,000 in western industrialized nations is a result of failure to breastfeed. The U.S. National Institute of Child Health and Human Development showed relative risk of SIDS for predominantly breastfed infants to be 0.2 for black infants and 0.27 for nonblack infants compared with that for babies formula-fed from birth (Harper & Hoffman, 1988).

Hypocalcemic Tetany

The high phosphate load in earlier formulas resulted in lower calcium retention in newborns and the depletion of infants' calcium levels, causing hypocalcemic tetany. Improved formulation has decreased this risk, but it still occurs.

Immune System Disorders

Artificial feeding may cause some of these immunologic phenomena associated with autoimmune diseases:

- Celiac disease (gluten sensitivity)—Formula feeding accelerates the development of Celiac disease (Auricchio et al., 1983).
- Crohn's disease—Formula feeding is a risk factor for Crohn's disease in adulthood (Rigas et al., 1993).
- Ulcerative colitis—Formula feeding is a risk factor for ulcerative colitis in adulthood (Rigas et al., 1993).

Chronic Liver Disease

Breastfeeding may have a role in preventing or modifying certain types of chronic liver disease; formula feeding may not offer this same protection.

---

*Source: Michael S. Kramer, MD (Professor, Departments of Pediatrics and of Epidemiology and Biostatistics, McGill University Faculty of Medicine, Montreal, Quebec, Canada): Controversy about the role of breastfeeding in preventing infection. *Breastfeeding Abstracts*, 11:2, 1991. Reprinted with permission from La Leche League International.

Insulin-Dependent Diabetes Mellitus

Two to 26% of cases of insulin-dependent diabetes mellitus (IDDM) are reported to be a result of formula feeding (Mayer et al., 1988). Formula feeding-induced IDDM results from an immunological attack on the pancreatic beta cells by bovine protein in genetically susceptible individuals. Breastfeeding, thus, may play a role in the prevention of IDDM (Samuelsson et al., 1993).

Allergies

Food allergies appear to be more frequent in formula-fed infants, with 7.4% of them developing cow's milk allergy (bovine proteins may be recognized as foreign) and up to 50% being allergic to soy (Cunningham et al., 1991). In 1989, the American Academy of Pediatrics (AAP) publicly stated that no published, well-controlled, double-blind studies exist to support the use of whey or casein hydrolysates for prophylaxis or treatment of infants with milk hypersensitivity. Anaphylactic reactions to both casein (Nutramigen, Alimentum, Pregestimil) and whey (Carnation Goodstart, Aifa-Re) hydrolysate formulas have been published (Businco et al., 1989; Ellis et al., 1991; Lifschitz et al., 1988; Saylor & Bahna, 1991; Schwartz & Amonette, 1991).

Breastfeeding may delay the development of atopic dermatitis (Chandra, 1987; Chandra et al., 1985); however, formula feeding increases instances of eczema and dermatitis. Altered levels of polyunsaturated fatty acids have been found in the milk of mothers whose infants have atopic eczema (Wright & Bolton, 1989). In infants infected with atopic eczema, the conversion of dietary linoleic acid to long-chain polyunsaturated metabolites is defective (Wright & Bolton, 1989). Gamma-linolenic acid helps alleviate the eczema (Biagi et al., 1988; Meigel et al., 1987; Morse et al., 1989). Human milk has γ-linolenic acid as a constituent. Infants with atopic dermatitis have been found to consume maternal milk with lower concentrations of a metabolite of linolenic acid (dihomo-γ-linolenic acid) (Morse et al., 1989). More on allergies can be found in Module 3, *The Science of Breastfeeding,* Chapter 2.

Lymphomas

There is a sixfold increase in childhood lymphomas in children who were formula-fed (Davis et al., 1988). Further, infants never breastfed or breastfed for less than two months were observed to be significantly less protected from Hodgkin's disease than those breastfed at least eight months (Schwartzbaum et al., 1991).

Miscellaneous Other Risks of Artificial Feeding

POTENTIAL FOR CONTAMINATION

Formula-fed infants are at risk of receiving contaminated formulas because of the following:

- Water supplies may be contaminated, resulting in diarrhea (each year 500 U.S. infants—ages 1 month to 4 years—die of diarrhea) and other symptoms of infection (Walker, 1993).
- Poorly educated families may prepare formula incorrectly because of an inability to read directions.
- Economically disadvantaged families may "water-down" formula in an effort to reduce cost. This can lead to water intoxication and reduced nutrient intake.
- Bacterial contamination may take place during production of formula or addition of water to reconstitute formula.

EXPERIMENTAL NATURE OF INGREDIENTS

Formula ingredients are regulated through the Infant Formula Act of 1980 which was created after 20,000 to 50,000 infants were exposed to chloride-deficient formulas in 1978 to 1979. This act has been instrumental in monitoring formula manufacturers (see Table 2B–1). The following are other examples of deficiencies and alterations over the years:

- Zinc-deficient formulas have caused retardation, inadequate growth, and skin lesions.
- Vitamin B_6-deficient formulas lead to seizures in infants.
- Marginal folic acid levels and the absence of vitamin C result in megaloblastic anemia.
- Protein amounts in infant formula may be 2.5 to 3 times greater than infants need. These high levels of protein are not known to offer advantages in terms of growth but they do place infants at a higher risk of developing hypernatremic dehydration during common situations of reduced water availability (decreased formula intake, high evaporative water losses from fever, or hot weather and diarrhea).

    Even though the levels of protein are higher, the necessary amino acids may not be available in formula. Until recently, formula did not contain taurine—an amino acid found in high levels in breastmilk. Formulas that have a 60:40 whey/casein ratio do not result in amino-acid profiles similar to those in breastfed infants yet they are promoted to be most like human milk.

    See Module 3, *The Science of Breastfeeding*, Chapter 2, for a more complete discussion of the differences in amino-acid profiles of breast versus formula-fed infants.

Table 2B–1   Recalls of Infant Formula Since 1982

Recall Class Number[a]	Date	Product[b]	Problem
I	1990	Soyalac Concentrated Infant Formula, 13-oz. cans (Loma Linda Foods)	Contaminated with heat-sensitive and heat-resistant bacteria
III	1989	Similac PM 60/40 powder, 16-oz., metal cans, low-iron infant formula (Ross Laboratories)	Deficient in vitamin D, below label claims for vitamin K
III	1989	Carnation Good Nature Infant Formula, 32-oz. containers, for babies over 6 months (Nestlé)	Unfit for food because of physical appearance; will not pass through an ordinary nipple
III	1989	Nutramigen Iron Fortified Protein Hydrolysate Formula, 4-oz. and 8-oz. bottles (Mead Johnson)	Deficient in vitamin D
III	1986	Soyalac Powder, 1.2-oz. foil pouches as physicians' samples (Loma Linda Foods)	Progressive vitamin A degradation
II	1986	SMA Ready-to-Feed, 32-oz. cans (Wyeth Laboratories)	Curdling, discoloration, off-color
II	1985	Gerber Meat Base Formula with Iron, 16-oz. cans of concentrated formula (Gerber)	Superpotent levels of vitamin A and subpotent levels of vitamin D
I	1985	Kama-Milk Powder, 6-oz. and 14-oz. cans (Kama Nutritional Products)	Marked in violation of the Infant Formula Act, deficient in folacin, vitamin D, and zinc
I	1985	Nutra-Milk Powder Infant Formula, 8-oz., 10-oz., and 16-oz. bottles (Kama Nutritional Products)	same as above
I	1985	Kama-Milk Powder Infant Formula, 14-oz. fiberboard cans, 14-oz. and 16-oz. bottles (Kama Nutritional Products)	same as above
I	1985	Pamphlet labeled in part "Edensoy," promotional material for Edensoy Soy Drinks (Eden Foods, Inc.)	Pamphlet erroneously suggests that Edensoy may be used as a substitute for human milk or infant formula
II	1985	Cow & Gate Improved Modified Infant Formula, 450-gm and 1-kg cans, U.S. Virgin Islands (Cow & Gate)	Deficient in copper and linoleic acid, not in compliance with Section 412 of Food, Drug and Cosmetic Act
III	1985	Lactogen Brand Infant Milk Formula in powder formula with iron, 227-gm, 450-gm, and 1,135-gm cans (Cow & Gate)	same as above
II	1985	5% glucose water in 4-oz. bottles (Ross Laboratories)	Glass particles in product caused by chipping of bottle necks
III	1984	Similac with Iron concentrate, 13-oz. (Ross Laboratories)	Overprocessed, resulting in the product becoming lumpy, brown, and unfit for consumption as food
II	1983	Soyalac Powder Milk-Free Fortified Soy Formula, 16-oz. cans (Loma Linda Foods)	Deficient in vitamin A
II	1983	Naturlac Infant Formula Powder, 22¾-oz. cans and trial-size 32-gm packets (Fillmore Foods)	Copper levels below minimum required by the Infant Formula Act; thiamine and vitamin B_6 less than stated on the label
I	1982	Nursoy Concentrated Liquid, 32-oz. cans; Nursoy Ready-to-Feed, 32-oz. cans (Wyeth Laboratories)	Deficient in vitamin B_6
I	1982	SMA Iron-Fortified Concentrated Liquid, 13-oz. cans; SMA Iron-Fortified Ready-to-Feed, 32-oz. cans; SMA Powder, 16-oz. cans; SMA E-Z Nurser Ready-to-Feed Nursettes (Wyeth Laboratories)	Deficient in vitamin B_6 (less than stated on the label)

[a]Class I Recall: A product that will cause serious health consequences or death when used.
Class II Recall: A product that may cause medically reversible health consequences when used.
Class III Recall: A product that is not likely to cause adverse health consequences when used.
[b]All data derived from the FDA Enforcement Report. Press Office, Food and Drug Administration, HFI-20, 5600 Fishers Lane, Rockville, MD 20857.

Source: Walker, M. (1993) A fresh look at the risks of artificial feeding. *J Hum Lact*, 9(2):107. Copyright © 1993, Human Sciences Press: New York. Reprinted with permission.

- Formula contains up to 20 times the iron in breastmilk (which is more readily absorbed). Iron is known to interfere with zinc and copper and may affect an infant's resistance to infection (Walker, 1993).
- Formula-fed infants were exposed to excessive concentrations of vitamin D in formulas in Maine, with samples containing >200% of the stated label claims for vitamin D (Walker, 1993).
- Formula nutrient recommendations are often based on data from adults or other species.

EXPOSURE TO CARCINOGENS AND ALLERGENS

Bottle nipples have contained carcinogens (nitrosides). Latex nipples may possibly cause allergic responses (Walker, 1993). Individuals with neural tube defects have been reported to have an increased sensitivity to latex.

RISKS FROM TYPE OF DELIVERY SYSTEM

Bottle feeding places infants at risk for the following:

- Possible apnea, bradycardia, and cyanosis caused by decreased TcO_2 tension and O_2 saturation resulting from the rapid flow rate allowed by artificial nipples (Mathew, 1988; Mathew, 1991; Meier, 1988).
- Bottles can be destructive to teeth (baby-bottle caries).
- Propping of bottles can lead to aspiration.

IMPAIRED SOCIAL INTERACTION

At times, caregivers will prop bottles instead of holding infants while they are being fed. This results in less contact between infants and caregivers, as well as missed opportunities for infants to develop social interaction skills.

IMPAIRED COGNITIVE SKILLS

Formula-fed infants have cognitive development delays and lower intelligence test scores. Developmental outcomes as measured by the Bayley Mental Development Index, the McCarthy Scales of Childrens' Abilities, and IQ testing have all shown that formula-fed infants have lower performance scores (Bauer et al., 1991; Lucas et al., 1992; Morley et al., 1988; Morrow-Tulcak et al., 1988; Taylor & Wadsworth, 1984).

EXCESSIVE COSTS

Infant formula is a 1.6-billion dollar a year market; the average family spends $500 to $1,200 per year on formula. The WIC program spends $500 million a year on formula (40% of all the formula sold in the United States). The increased number of infections from formula feeding result in increased health-care costs (see Table 2B–2).

Table 2B-2   Infant Feeding Costs[1]

Savings	Cost/Year[2]	Annual Savings If Breastfed
Breastfeeding (500 kcal/day)	$298	—
Formula[3]		
Powder, 1-lb. can	$664	$366
Concentrate, 13-oz. can	$804	$506
Ready-to-feed, 32-oz. can	$981	$683
Ready-to-feed, 6 pack (8-oz. cans)	$1,523	$1,225
Nursette[4]		
8-oz. bottles (8 pack)	$2,196	$1,898
6-oz. bottles (8 pack)	$2,607	$2,309
4-oz. bottles (8 pack)	$3,369	$3,071

[1] Data from San Diego, 1991.

[2] Formula costs/year based on average recommended formula intake for the first year of life of 9,634.21 fl. oz.

[3] Formula cost based on supermarket shelf price of Similac (Ross Laboratories).

[4] Formula cost based on supermarket shelf price of Enfamil (Mead-Johnson).

Source: Distributed at the International Lactation Consultant Association Annual Meeting, Scottsdale, AZ, 1993.

Importance of Informed Decision Making

The advocacy of breastfeeding has been cited by the United Nations Children Fund as the most crucial factor for the protection of children in the decades ahead. Many major organizations have joined the United Nations in pronouncing breastfeeding's unique properties to the international community.

In many nations, formula-fed infants get far more illnesses and are 25 times more likely to die in childhood than those exclusively breastfed for six months. Breastmilk provides more than just nutrition. Breastmilk provides live cells that cannot be reproduced and that convey factors to prime the immune system and impact on the establishment of gut integrity.

Health-care professionals and laymen alike now know that breastmilk is the best choice for every baby; yet, we still question whether breastfeeding is the best choice for every mother. Formula feeding has become so much a way of life that few parents and professionals are aware of the risks of artificial feeding. Concerns over health-care professionals inducing guilt has been giving them a reason not to inform families of the vast differences between infant-feeding methods.

Professionals rally around informed consent for every other health-care decision patients must make. Parents have a right to know the consequences of a decision and withholding information will generate more anger than guilt. Parents must be informed of the risks of artificial feeding so they can weigh the benefits and risks associated with different feeding methods for themselves.

POST-TEST

For questions 1 to 7, choose the best answer.

1. Formula feeding is associated with

    A. decreased risk of childhood lymphoma.
    B. decreased atopic dermatitis.
    C. increased stooling.
    D. increased risk of IDDM.

2. Formula feeding offers a means for

    A. infants to receive an excessive amount of protein.
    B. poorly educated families to correctly feed their infant.
    C. protection against bacterial contamination.
    D. economically disadvantaged families to inexpensively feed their infants.

3. Chance is a potential source of negative results in research because of

    A. an increase in statistical power.
    B. inadequate statistical power.
    C. an increase in sample size.
    D. selection bias.

4. Formula feeding exposes infants to

    A. increased forms of facial muscle exercises.
    B. optimal levels of bioavailable nutrients.

    C. low renal solute loads.

    D. increased risk of contamination.

5. The magnitude of the protective effect

    A. is larger in developing countries than in developed countries.

    B. is larger in developed countries than in developing countries.

    C. is smaller in developing countries than in developed countries.

    D. is no different between developed and developing countries.

6. Risk factors for SIDS include:

    A. maternal smoking, prone sleeping position, not breastfeeding.

    B. maternal smoking, not breastfeeding, not drinking.

    C. not drinking, maternal smoking, prone sleeping position.

    D. not breastfeeding, not smoking, not drinking.

7. Poverty, regardless of whether a nation is considered developed or developing, yields:

    A. increased housing opportunities.

    B. lack of sanitation and potable water.

    C. hygienic conditions.

    D. heavy exposure to microbes.

For questions 8 to 10, choose the best answer from the following key:

    A. if response 1, 2, and 3 are correct.   **D. if only 4 is correct.**

    B. if responses 1 and 3 are correct.   **E. if all are correct.**

    C. if responses 2 and 4 are correct.

8. Which of the following are hazards of formula feeding?

    1. Formula composition alters during shelf life.

    2. Formula feeding may expose infants to carcinogens and allergens.

    3. Formula-fed infants have lower cognitive development.

    4. Formula is composed of living cells and antibodies.

9. Which of the following is a risk of formula feeding?

    1. Increased risk of chronic liver disease

    2. Increased number of infants with allergies

    3. Increased likelihood of developing necrotizing enterocolitis

    4. Increased protection against infection

10. The experimental nature of formula ingredients results or has resulted in

    1. infants being exposed to a chloride-deficient formula.

    2. a vitamin B_6-deficiency that caused seizures in some infants.

    3. high amounts of protein that place infants at risk of hypernatremic dehydration.

    4. infants receiving up to 20 times the amount of iron in breastmilk.

For questions 11 to 16, choose the best answer.

11. Formula-fed infants are less likely than breastfed infants to

    A. be protected against respiratory infection.

    B. develop infant botulism.

    C. become insulin-dependent diabetics.

    D. be hospitalized during their first four months of life.

12. Formula ingredients are regulated through the

    A. Infant Nutritional Support Act of 1970.
    B. Infant Feeding Act of 1980.
    C. Formula Regulatory Act of 1970.
    D. Infant Formula Act of 1980.

13. _____ is caused by the high phosphate loads in formula, causing twitching, convulsions, and atypical seizures.

    A. Hypocalcemic tetany
    B. SIDS
    C. Chronic liver disease
    D. Elevated renal solute load

14. Formula feeding

    A. increases the risk of necrotizing enterocolitis in infants born at less than thirty-weeks gestation.
    B. decreases the risk of recurrent otitis media.
    C. decreases the risk of morbidity and mortality.
    D. imposes a four- to sixfold lower risk of influenza bacteremia.

15. Botulism resulting in sudden death

    A. occurs in both breast- and formula-fed infants.
    B. occurs only in formula-fed infants.
    C. occurs in weaning breastfed infants.
    D. occurs in breastfed infants.

16. Formula feeding has been shown to

    A. decrease the intensity of infection in the infant.
    B. lower the incidence of infection in the infant.
    C. prolong the duration of infection in the infant.
    D. solely protect the infant's gastrointestinal tract from infection.

For questions 17 to 20, choose from the following key:

   A. Increased by formula feeding
   B. Decreased by formula feeding

17. Necrotizing enterocolitis in preterm infants

18. Severity of respiratory synctial virus

19. Renal solute load

20. *H. influenzae* bacteremia

References

Ahmed, F, Clemens, JD, Rao, MR, Khan, MR, Haque, E (1992). Community-based evaluation of the effect of breastfeeding on the risk of microbiologically confirmed or clinically presumptive shigellosis in Bangladeshi children. *Pediatrics*, 90(3):406-11.

Albertson, BD (1989). Constituents of saliva and breastmilk. *Int J Gyn Obste*, 1(Suppl):53-65.

American Academy of Pediatrics (AAP), Committee on Nutrition (1989). Hypoallergenic infant formulas. *Pediatrics* 83:1068-69.

American Academy of Pediatrics, Committee on Nutrition (1992). The use of whole cow's milk in infancy. *Pediatrics*, 89:1105-9.

Ashraf, RN, Jalil, F, Zaman, S, Karlberg, J, Khan, SR, Lindblad, BS, Hanson, LA (1991). Breastfeeding and protection against neonatal sepsis in a high-risk population. *Arch Dis Child*, 66(4):488-90.

Auricchio, S (1983). Gluten-sensitive enteropathy and infant nutrition. *J Pediatr Gastroenterol Nutr*, 2(suppl 1): S304-09.

Auricchio, S, Follo, D, de Ritis, G, Giunta, A, Marzorati, D, Prampolini, L, Ansaldi, N, Levi, P, Dall'olio, D, Bossi, A, et al. (1983). Does breastfeeding protect against the development of clinical symptoms of celiac disease in children? *J Pediatr Gastroenterol Nutr*, 2(3):428-33.

Axelsson, I, Jakobsson, I, Lindberg, T, Polberger, S, Benediktsson, B, Raiha, N (1989). Macromolecular absorption in preterm and term infants. *Acta Paediatr Scand*, 78:532-37.

Barros, FC, Victoria, CG, Vaughan, JP (1986). Breastfeeding and socioeconomic status in Southern Brazil. *Acta Paediatr Scand*, 75(4):558-62.

Bauchner, H, Leventhal, JM, Shapiro, ED (1986). Studies of breastfeeding and infections: How good is the evidence? *JAMA*, 256:887-92.

Bauer, G, Ewald, S, Hoffman, J, et al. (1991). Breastfeeding and cognitive development of three-year-old children. *Psychol Rep*, 68:12-18.

Biagi, PL, Bordoni, A, Masi, M, Ricci, G, Fanelli, C, Patrizi, A, Ceccolino, E (1988). A long-term study of the use of evening primrose oil (Efamol) in atopic children. *Drugs Exp Clin Res*, 14:285-90.

Birch, E, et al. (1993). Breastfeeding and optimal visual development. *J Pediatr Ophthalmol Strab*, 30(1):33-38.

Blackberg, L, Hernell, O (1993). Bile salt–stimulated lipase in human milk: Evidence that bile salt induces lipid binding and activation via binding to different sites. *FEBS Lett*, 323(3):207-10.

Bocar, D (1993). *Breastfeeding Educator Program*. Lactation Consultant Services: Oklahoma City, OK.

Briend, A, Wojtyniak, B, Rowland, MGM (1988). Breastfeeding, nutritional state and child survival in rural Bangladesh. *Br Med J*, 296:879-82.

Brines, RD, Brock, JH (1983). The effect of trypsin and chymotrypsin on the in vitro antimicrobial and iron-binding properties of lactoferrin in human milk and bovine colostrum. *Biochim Biophys Acta*, 759:229-35.

Brown, KH, Black, RE, Romana, GL, Kanashiro, HC (1989). Infant-feeding practices and their relationship with diarrheal and other diseases in Huascar (Lima), Peru. *Pediatrics*, 83:31-40.

Bryant, C, Roy, M (1989). *Best Start Training Manual*. Best Start: Tampa.

Bullen, JJ, Rogers, HJ, Griffiths, E (1978). Role of iron in bacterial infection. *Curr Top Microbiol Immunol*, 80: 1-35.

Buranasin, B (1991). The effects of rooming-in on the success of breastfeeding and the decline in abandonment of children. *Asia Pac J Pub Health*, 5(3):217-20.

Businco, L, Cantani, A, Longhi, MA, et al. (1989). Anaphylactic reactions to a cow's milk whey protein hydrolysate (Alfa-Re, Nestlé) in infants with cow's milk allergy. *Ann Allergy*, 62:333-35.

Butte, NF, Garza, C, Johnson, CA, et al. (1984). Longitudinal changes in milk composition of mothers delivering preterm and term infants. *Early Hum Dev*, 9:153-62.

131

Butte, NF, Garza, C (1986). Anthropometry in the appraisal of lactation performance among well-nourished women. In: Hamosh, M, Goldman, AS (Eds), *Human Lactation 2: Maternal and Environmental Factors* (pp. 61-67). Plenum Press: New York.

Caplan, MS, Sun, XM, Hsueh, W, Hageman, JR (1990). Role of platelet-activating factor and tumor necrosis factor—alpha in neonatal necrotizing enterocolitis. *J Pediatr*, 116:960-64.

Chandra, RK (1982). Physical growth of exclusively breast-fed infants. *Nutr Res*, 2:275-76.

Chandra, RK (1987). Prevention of atopic disease: environmental engineering utilizing antenatal antigen avoidance and breastfeeding. In: Goldman, AS, Atkinson, SA, Hanson, LA (Eds), *Human Lactation 3: The Effects of Human Milk on the Recipient Infants* (pp. 269-74). Plenum Press: New York.

Chandra, RK, Puri, S, Cheema, PS (1985). Predictive value of cord blood IgE in the development of atopic disease and role of breastfeeding in its prevention. *Clin Allergy*, 15:517-22.

Chen, Y, Shunzhang, Y, Wan-xian, L (1988). Artificial feeding and hospitalization in the first eighteen months of life. *Pediatrics*, 81:58-62.

Chipman, DM, Sharon, N (1969). Mechanism of lysozyme action. *Science*, 165:454-65.

Clemens, JD, Stanton, B, Stoll, B, Shahid, NS, Banu, H, Chowdhury, AKMA (1986). Breastfeeding as a determinant of severity in shigellosis: Evidence for protection throughout the first three years of life in Bangladeshi children. *Am J Epidemiol*, 123:710-20.

Cochi, S L, Fleming, DW, Hightower, AW, Limpakarnjanarat, K, Facklam, RR, Smith, JD, Sikes, RK, Broome, CV (1986). Primary invasive *Haemophilus influenzae* type B disease: A population-based assessment of risk factors. *J Pediatr*, 108:887-96.

Cunningham, AS (1988). Meta-analysis and methodology review: What's in a name? *J Pediatr*, 113(2):328-29.

Cunningham, AS (1989). Pig roasts, science and babies: A reply to Leventhal, Shapiro and Bauchner. *J Hum Lact*, 5(3):128-30.

Cunningham, AS, Jelliffe, DB, Jelliffe, EF (1991). Breastfeeding and health in the 1980s: A global epidemiologic review. *J Pediatr*, 118(5):659-66.

Czajka-Narins, DM, Jung, E (1986). Physical growth of breast-fed and formula-fed infants from birth to age two years. *Nutr Res*, 6:753-62.

Davis, MK, Savitz, DA, Graubard, BI (1988). Infant feeding and childhood cancer. *Lancet*, 2:365-68.

DeCurtis, M, Paone, C, Vetrano, G, Romano, G, Paludetto, R, Ciccimarra, F (1987). A case control study of necrotizing enterocolitis occurring over eight years in a neonatal intensive care unit. *Eur J Pediatr*, 146:398-400.

de Duran, CM, Assayas, R, Sanchez de Gonalez, L (1991). Cytologic diagnosis of milk microaspiration. *Immunol Allergy Practice*, xiii(10):402-5.

Deutsch, H (1945). *The Psychology of Women, Volume Two: Motherhood*. Grune & Stratton: New York.

Dewey, KG, Heinig, MJ, Nommsen, LA (1993). Maternal weight-loss patterns during prolonged lactation. *Am J Clin Nutr*, 91:867-72.

Dewey, KG, Heinig, MJ, Nommsen, LA, Lönnerdal, B (1989). Infant growth and breastfeeding. *Am J Clin Nutr*, 50:1116-17.

Dewey, KG, Heinig, MJ, Nommsen, LA, Lönnerdal, B (1990). Growth patterns of breastfed infants during the first year of life: The DARLING study. In: Atkinson, SA, Hanson, LA, Chandra, R (Eds), *Human Lactation 4: Breastfeeding Nutrition, Infection and Infant Growth in Developed and Emerging Countries* (pp. 269-82). ARTS Biomedical Publishers: St. John's, Newfoundland, Canada.

Dewey, KG, Heinig, MJ, Nommsen, LA, Lönnerdal, B (1991). Maternal versus infant factors related to breast-milk intake and residual milk volume: The DARLING study. *Pediatrics*, 87(6):829-37.

Dewey, KG, Lönnerdal, B (1983). Milk and nutrient intake of breastfed infants from 1 to 6 months: Relation to growth and fatness. *J Pediatr Gastroenterol Nutr*, 2:497-506.

Duffy, LC, Byers, TE, Riepenhoff-Talty, M, La Scolea, LJ, Zielezny, MA, Ogra, PL (1986a). The effects of infant feeding on rotavirus-induced gastroenteritis: A prospective study. *Am J Pub Health*, 76:259-63.

Duffy, LC, Riepenhoff-Talty, M, Ogra, PL, Byers, TE, La Scolea, LJ, Zielezny, MA, Dryja, DM (1986b). Modulation of rotavirus enteritis during breastfeeding. *Am J Dis Child*, 140:1164-68.

Duffy, LC, Zielezny, MA, Dryja, D, Faden, H, Ogra, PL (1992). *Bifidobacterium* Colonization of Human Intestine: Cultivation and Characterization of Resident and Ingestion Strains. In: Picciano, MF, Lönnerdal, B (Eds), *Mechanisms Regulating Lactation and Infant Nutrient Utilization* (pp. 383-87). Wiley-Liss: New York.

Duncan, B, Ey, J, Holberg, CJ, Wright, AL, Martinez, FD, Taussing, LM (1993). Exclusive breast-feeding for at least four months protects against otitis media. *Pediatrics*, 91(5): 867-72.

Duncan, B, Schaefer, C, Sibley, B, Fonseca, NM (1984). Reduced growth velocity in exclusively breastfed infants. *Am J Dis Child*, 138:309-13.

Dusdieker, LB, Hemingway, DL, Stumbo, PJ (1994). Is milk production impaired by dieting during lactation? *Am J Clin Nutr*, 59(4):833-40.

Editorial (1986). Infant botulism. *Lancet*, 2:1256-57.

Eibl, MM, Wolf, HM, Furnkranz, H, Rosenkranz, A (1988). Prevention of necrotizing enterocolitis in low-birthweight infants by IgA-IgG feeding. *N Engl J Med*, 319: 1-7.

Elk, J, Magnus E (1982). Plasma and red cell folate values and folate requirements in formula-fed term infants. *J Pediatr*, 100:738-44.

Ellis, MH, Short, JA, Heiner, DC (1991). Anaphylaxis after ingestion of a recently introduced whey protein formula. *J Pediatr*, 118:74-77.

Facione, N (1990). Otitis media: An overview of acute and chronic disease. *Nurse Pract*, 15:11-22.

Faden, H, Stanievich, J, Brodsky, L, Berstein, J, Ogra, PL (1990). Changes in nasopharyngeal flora during otitis media of childhood. *Pediatr Infect Dis J,* 9(9):623-26.

Faden, H, Waz, MJ, Bernstein, JM, Brodsky, L, Stanievich, J, Ogra, PL (1991). Nasopharyngeal flora in the first three years of life in normal and otitis-prone children. *Ann Otol Rhinol Laryngol,* 199(8):612-15.

Feachem, RG, Koblinsky, MA (1984). Interventions for the control of diarrheal diseases among young children: Promotion of breastfeeding. *Bull WHO,* 62:271-91.

Finberg, L (1989). Comment by Finberg, *J Nutr,* 119:1788.

Fomon, SJ (Ed) (1993). *Nutrition of Normal Infants.* Mosby: St. Louis.

Forsum, E. Sadurskis, A (1986). Growth, body composition and breastmilk intake of Swedish infants during early life. *Early Hum Dev,* 14:121-29.

Fosarelli, PP, De Angelis, C, Winkelstein, J, Mellitis, ED (1985). Infectious illnesses in the first two years of life. *Pediatr Infect Dis J,* 4:153-59.

Friss, HE, Rubin, LG, Carsons, S, Baranowski, J, Lipsitz, PJ (1988). Plasma fibronectin concentrations in breast-fed and formula-fed neonates. *Arch Dis Child,* 63:528-32.

Furukawa, M, Narahara, H, Yasuda, K, Johnson, JM (1993). Presence of platelet-activating factor—acetylhydrolase in milk. *J Lip Res,* 34:1603-9.

Gabbe, S (1991). *Obstetrics—Normal and Problem Pregnancies.* Churchill Livingston: New York.

Garza, C, et al. (1987a). Special properties of human milk, *Clin Perinatol,* 14:11-31.

Garza, C, Stuff, J, Butte, N (1987b). Growth of the breast-fed infant. In: Goldman, AS, Atkinson, SA, Hanson, LA (Eds), *Human Lactation 3: The Effects of Human Milk on the Recipient Infants.* Plenum Press: New York.

Gendrel, D, Richard-Lenoble, D , Kombila, M., Baziomo, JM, Gendrel, C, Nardou, M (1988). Breastfeeding and intestinal parasites [French]. *Archives Francaises de Pediatrie,* 45(6):399-404.

Gendrel, D, Richard-Lenoble, D, Kombila, M, Gendrel, C, Baziomo, J (1989). *Giardiasis* and breastfeeding in urban Africa. *Pediatr Infect Dis J,* 8:58-59.

Goldman, AS, et al. (1986). Anti-inflammatory properties of human milk, *Acta Paediatr Scand,* 75:689-95.

Goldman, AS, Goldblum, RM (1989). Immunologic system in human milk: Characteristics and effects. In: Lebenthal, E (Ed), *Textbook of Gastroenterology and Nutrition in Early Infancy,* 2nd ed (pp. 135-42). Raven Press: New York.

Goldman, AS, Goldblum, RM, Hanson, LA (1991). Anti-inflammatory systems in human milk. *Adv Exp Med Biol,* 262:69-76.

Goldman, AS, Thorpe, LW, Goldblum, RM, Hanson, LA (1986). Anti-inflammatory properties of human milk. *Acta Paediatr Scand,* 75:689-95.

Grillner, L, Broberger, U, Chrystie, I, Ransjo, U (1985). Rotavirus infections in newborns: An epidemiological and clinical study. *Scand J Infect Dis,* 17:349-55.

Gyllenberg, H, Roine, P (1957). The value of colony counts in evaluating the abundance of *"Lactobacillus" bifidus* in infant faeces. *Acta Pathol Microbiol Scand,* 41:144.

Gyorgy, P, Jeanloz, RW, von Nicolai, H, Zilliken, F (1974). Undialyzable growth factors for *Lactobacillus bifidus var. Pennsylvanicus*: Protective effect of sialic acid bound to glycoproteins and oligosaccharids against bacterial degradation. *Eur J Biochem,* 43:29-33.

Habicht, JP, Da Vanzo, J, Butz, WP (1986). Does breast-feeding really save lives, or are apparent benefits due to biases? *Am J Epidemiol,* 123:279-90.

Haddock, RL, Cousens, SN, Guzman, CC (1991). Infant diet and salmonellosis. *Am J Public Health,* 81(8):997-1000.

Hahn-Zoric, M, et al. (1990). Antibody responses to parenteral and oral vaccines are impaired by conventional and low-protein formulas as compared to breastfeeding. *Acta Paediatr Scand,* 79:1137-42.

Hallman, M, Bry, K, Hopper, K, et al. (1992). Inositol supplementation in premature infants with respiratory distress syndrome. *N Engl J Med,* 326:1233-39.

Hamosh, M (1989). Enzymes in human milk: Their role in nutrient digestion, gastrointestinal function and nutrient delivery to the newborn infant. In: Lebenthal, E (Ed), *Textbook of Gastroenterology and Nutrition in Early Infancy,* 2nd ed, Raven Press: New York.

Hanson, LA, Ashraf, R, Zamar, S, Karlberg, J, Lindblad, BS, Jalil, F (1994). Breastfeeding is a natural contraceptive and prevents disease and death in infants, linking infant mortality and birth rates. *Acta Paediatr,* 83:3-6.

Hanson, LA, Bergstrom, S (1990). The link between infant mortality and birth rates—the importance of breastfeeding as a common factor. *Acta Paediatr Scand,* 79:481-89.

Hanson, LA, Lindquist, B, Hofvander, Y, Zetterstrom, R (1985). Breastfeeding as a protection against gastroenteritis and other infections. *Acta Paediatr Scand,* 74:641-42.

Harabuchi, Y, Faden, H, Yamanaka, N, Duffy, L, Wolf, J, Krystofik, D (1994). Human milk secretory IgA antibody to nontypeable *Haemophilus influenzae*: Possible protective effects against nasopharyngeal colonization. *J Pediatr,* 124:193-98.

Harper, RM, Hoffman, HJ (Eds) (1988). *Sudden Infant Death Syndrome: Risk Factors and Basic Mechanisms* (pp. 197-201, 226-227, 503). PMA Publishing Corp.: New York.

Hitchcock, NE, Coy, JF (1989). The growth of healthy Australian infants in relation to infant feeding and social group. *Med J Austr,* 150:306-11.

Hitchcock, NE, Gracey, M, Galmour, AI (1985). The growth of breastfed and artificially fed infants from birth to twelve months. *Acta Paediatr Scand,* 74:240-45.

Holmgren, J, Svennerholm, AM, Ahren, C (1981). Nonimmunoglobulin fraction of human milk inhibits bacterial adhesion (hemagglutination) and enterotoxin binding of *Escherichiae cole* and *Vibrio cholerae. Infect Immun,* 33:136-41.

Howie, PW, Forsyth, JS, Ogston, SA, Clark, A, Florey, C (1990). Protective effect of breastfeeding against infections. *Br Med J,* 300:11-16.

IBFAN/IOCU (1990). *Protecting Infant Health—A Health Worker's Guide to the International Code of Marketing of Breast Milk Substitutes,* 6th ed. IBFAN/IOCU: Penang, Malaysia.

Institute of Medicine (IOM) (1991). *Nutrition During Lactation.* National Academy Press: Washington.

International Lactation Consultant Association Annual Meeting (1993). *Infant Feeding Costs,* Scottsdale, AZ.

Istre, GR, Compton, R, Novotny, T (1986). Infant botulism: Three cases in a small town. *Am J Dis Child,* 140: 1013-14.

Jayashree, S, Bhan, MH, Raj, P, Kumar, R, Svenssan, L, Stintzing, C, Bhandan, N (1988). Neonatal rotavirus infection and its relation to cord blood antibodies. *Scand J Infect Dis,* 20:249-53.

Jensen, RG (1989). Lipids in human milk—composition and fat-soluble vitamins. In: Lebenthal, E (Ed), *Textbook of Gastroenterology and Nutrition in Early Infancy,* 2nd ed (pp. 157-208). Raven Press: New York.

Keller, MA, Kidd, RM, Bryson, YJ, Turner, JL, Carter, J (1981). Lymphokine production by human milk lymphocytes. *Infect Immun,* 32:632-36.

Keun-Young, Y, Tajima, K, Kuroishi, T, et al. (1992). Independent protective effect of lactation against breast cancer: A case-control study in Japan. *Am J Epidemiol,* 135: 726-33.

Khan, SR, Jalil, F, Zaman, S, Lindblad, BS, Karlberg, J (1993). Early child health in Lahore, Pakistan: X Mortality. *Acta Paediatr,* 82(390, suppl):109-17.

Kirkpatrick, CH, et al. (1971). Inhibition of growth of *Candida albicans* by iron-unsaturated lactoferrin: Relation to host defense mechanisms in chronic mucocutaneous candidiasis. *J Infect Dis,* 124:539.

Kohl, S, Pickering, LK, Cleary, TG, Steinmentz, KD, Loo, LS (1980). Human colostral cytotoxicity. II: Relative defects in colostral leukocyte cytotoxicity and inhibition of peripheral blood leukocyte cytotozicity by colostrum. *J Infect Dis,* 142:884-91.

Koldovsky, O, Bedrick, A, Rao, RK (1989). Physiological functions of human milk hormones. *Acta Paediatr Scand,* 351(suppl):94-96.

Koletzko, S, Sherman, P, Corey, M, et al. (1989). Role of infant feeding practices in development of Crohn's disease in childhood. *Br Med J,* 298(6688):1617-18.

Kramer, M (1991). Controversy about the role of breastfeeding in preventing infection. *Breastfeeding Abstr,* 11:2.

Labbok, MH (1989). *Breastfeeding and Fertility. Mothers and Children,* 8(1, suppl). American Public Health Association: Washington.

Labbok, MH, Hendershot, GE (1987). Does breast-feeding protect against malocclusion? An analysis of the 1981 Child Health Supplement to the National Health Interview Survey. *Am J Prev Med,* 3:227-32.

Lanner, LJ, Habicht, JP, Kardjati, S (1990). Breastfeeding protects infants in Indonesia against illness and weight loss due to illness. *Am J Epidemiol,* 131:322-31.

Lawton, JWM, Shortridge, KF, Wong, RLC, Ng, MH (1979). Interferon synthesis by human colostral leucocytes. *Arch Dis Child,* 54:127-30.

Leventhal, JM, Shapiro, ED, Aten CB, et al. (1986). Does breastfeeding protect against infections in infants less than three months of age? *Pediatrics,* 78:896-903.

Lewis, P, et al. (1991). The resumption of ovulation and menstruation in well-nourished population of women breastfeeding for an extended period of time. *Fertil Steril,* 55(3):529-36.

Leyva-Cobian, F, Clemente, J (1984). Phenotypic characterization and functional activity of human milk macrophages. *Immunol Lett,* 8:249-56.

Lifschitz, CH, Hawkins, HK, Guerra, C, et al. (1988). Anaphylactic shock due to cow's milk protein hypersensitivity in a breastfed infant. *J Pediatr Gastroenterol Nutr,* 7:141-44.

Lucas, A, Cole, TJ (1990). Breastmilk and neonatal necrotizing enterocolitis. *Lancet,* 336, 1519-23.

Lucas, A, Morley R, Cole, TJ, et al. (1992). Breastmilk and subsequent intelligence quotient in children born preterm. *Lancet,* 339:261-64.

Macedo, CG (1988). Infant mortality in the Americas. *PAHO Bull,* 22:303-12.

Manning-Dalton, C, Allen, LH (1983). The effects of lactation on energy and protein consumption, postpartum weight change and body composition of well-nourished North American women. *Nutr Res,* 3:293-308.

Mata, L (1982). Breastfeeding, diarrheal disease and malnutrition in less developed countries. In: Lifshitz, F (Ed), *Pediatric Nutrition, Infant Feedings: Deficiencies, Decreases* (pp. 355-72). Marcel Dekker: New York.

Mathew, O (1988). Respiratory control during nipple feeding in preterm infants. *Pediatr Pulmonol,* 5:220-24.

Mathew, O (1991). Breathing patterns of preterm infants during bottlefeeding: Role of milk flow. *J Pediatr,* 119: 960-65.

Mayer, EJ, Hamman, RF, Gay, EC, et al. (1988). Reduced risk of IDDM among breastfed children. *Diabetes,* 37:1625-32.

Meier, P (1988). Bottle-and breast-feeding effects on transcutaneous oxygen pressure and temperature in preterm infants. *Nurs Res,* 37:36-41.

Meigel, W, Dettke, T, Meigel, EM, Lenze, V (1987). Additional oral treatment of atopic dermatitis with unsaturated fatty acids. *Z Hautkr,* 62(suppl 1):100-103.

Menard, D, Arsenault, P (1988). Epidermal and neural growth factors in milk: Effects of epidermal growth factor on the development of the gastrointestinal tract. In: Nestlé Nutrition Workshop Series, *Biology of Human Milk* (pp. 15:105-22). Raven Press: New York.

Mitchell, EA, Scragg, R, Stewart, AW, Becroft, DMO, Taylor, BJ, Ford, RPK, Hassall, IB, Barry, DMJ, Allen, EM, Roberts, AP (1991). Cot death supplement: Results from the first year of the New Zealand cot death study. *NZ Med J,* 104:71-76.

Morley, R, Cole, TJ, Powell, R, et al. (1988). Mother's choice to provide breastmilk and developmental outcome. *Arch Dis Child,* 63:1382-85.

Morrow-Tlucak, M, Houde, RH, Ernhart, CB (1988). Breastfeeding and cognitive development in the first two years of life. *Soc Sci Med,* 26:635-39.

Morse, PF, Horrobin, DF, Manku, MS, et al. (1989). Meta-analysis of placebo-controlled studies of the efficacy of Epogam in the treatment of atopic exzema: Relationship between plasma-essential fatty acid changes and clinical response. *Br J Dermatol,* 121:75-90.

National Research Council (NRC) (1989). *Recommended Dietary Allowances.* National Academy Press: Washington, DC.

Nelson, SE, Rogers, RP, Ziegler, EE, Fomon, SJ (1989). Gain in weight and length during early infancy. *Early Hum Dev,* 19:223-39.

Newcomb, PA (1994). Lactation and a reduced risk of premeneopausal cancer. *N Engl J Med,* 330:81-87.

Otnaess, AB, Svennerholm, AM (1982). Non-immunoglobulin fraction of human milk protects rabbits against enterotoxin-induced intestinal fluid secretion. *Infect Immunol,* 35:738-40.

Otnaess, AB, Laegreid, A, Ertresvag, K (1983). Inhibition of enterotoxin from *Escherichia coli* and *Vibrio cholerae* by gangliosides from human milk *Infect Immunol,* 40:563-69.

Orloff, SL, Wallingford, JC, McDougal, JS (1993). Inactivation of human immunodeficiency virus Type I in human milk: Effects of intrinsic factors in human milk and of pasteurization. *J Hum Lact,* 9:13-19.

Palmer, G (1988). *The Politics of Breastfeeding.* Pandora Press: London.

Pape, JW, Levine, E, Beaulieu, ME, et al. (1987). Cryptosporidiosis in Haitian children. *Am J Trop Med Hyg,* 36:333-37.

Patton, S (1994). Detection of large fragments of the human milk mucin-1 in feces of breastfed infant. *J Pediatr Gastroenterol Nutr,* 18(2):225-30.

Pereira, GR, Baker, L, Egler J, et al. (1990). Serum myoinositol concentrations in premature infants fed human milk, formula for infants, and parenteral nutrition. *Am J Clin Nutr,* 51:589-93.

Picciano, MF, Guthrie, HA (1976). Copper, iron, and zinc contents of mature human milk. *Am J Clin Nutr,* 29:242-54.

Pisacane, A, Graziano, L, Mazzarella, G, et al. (1992). Breast-feeding and urinary tract infection. *J Pediatr,* 120:87-89.

Pollack, RF, Koldovsky, O, Nishioka, K (1992). Polyamines in human and rat milk and in infant formulas. *Am J Clin Nutr,* 56(2):371-75.

Porro, E, Antognoni, G, Midulla, F, et al. (1988). *Breastfeeding and Bronchiolitis.* Ambulatory Pediatric Association Program book, Chicago.

Prentice, A, et al. (1989). Breast-milk IgA & lactoferrin survival in the gastrointestinal tract—a study in rural Gambian children. *Acta Paediatr Scand,* 78: 505-12.

Pukander, J, Luotonen, J, Timonen, M, Karma, P (1985). Risk factors affecting the occurrence of acute otitis media among 2–3-year-old urban children. *Acta Otolaryngol,* 100:260-65.

Putnam, JC., Carlson, SE, DeVoe, PW, Barness, LA (1982). The effect of variations in dietary fatty acids on the fatty acid composition of erythrocyte phosphatidylcholine and phosphatidylethanolamine in human infants. *Am J Clin Nutr,* 36(1):106-14.

Rassin, DK, Sturman, JA, Gaull, GE (1978). Taurine and other free amino acids and breast milk of vegans compared with omnivores. *Br J Nutr,* 56:17-27.

Resta, S, Luby, JP, Rosenfeld, CR, Siegel, JD (1985). Isolation and propagation of a human enteric coronavirus. *Science,* 229(4717):978-81.

Rigas, A, Rigas, B, Glassman, M, et al. (1993). Breast-feeding and maternal smoking in the etiology of Crohn's disease and ulcerative colitis in childhood. *Ann Epidemiol,* 3:387-92.

Rogan, WJ (1989). Cancer from PCBs in breastmilk? A risk benefit analysis [Abstract No. 612]. *Pediatr Res,* 25:105A.

Rogan, WJ, Gladen BC, McKinney, JD, Carreras, N, Hardy, P, Thullen, J, Tinglestadt, J, Tully, M (1987). Polychlorinated biphenyls (PCBs) and dichlorophenyl dichloroethene (DDE) in human milk: Effects on growth, morbidity and duration of lactation. *Am J Pub Health,* 77:1294-97.

Ruiz-Palacios, GM, Lopez-Vidal, Y, Galva, J, Cleary, TG, Pickering, LK (1986). Impact of breastfeeding on diarrhea prevention. *Pediatr Res,* 20:320A.

Saarinen, UM, Siimes, MA (1979). Role of prolonged breast feeding in infant growth. *Acta Paediatr Scand,* 68:245-50.

Salmenpera, L, Perheentupa, J, Pakarinen, P, Siimes, MA (1986). Cu nutrition in infants during prolonged exclusive breastfeeding: Low intake but rising serum concentrations of Cu and ceruloplasmin. *Am J Clin Nutr,* 43:251-57.

Salmenpera, l, Perheentupa, J, Siimes, MA (1985). Exclusively breast-fed healthy infants grow slower than reference infants. *Pediatr Res,* 19:307-12.

Samson, RR, Mirtle, C, McClelland, DBL (1980). The effect of digestive enzymes on the binding and bacteriostatic properties of lactoferrin and vitamin B_{12} binder in human milk. *Acta Paediatr Scand,* 69:517-23.

Samuelsson, U, Johansson, C, Ludvigsson, J (1993). Breastfeeding seems to play a marginal role in the prevention of insulin-dependent diabetes mellitus. *Diabetes Res Clin Pract,* 82:314-19.

Saylor, J, Bahna, S (1991). Anaphylaxis to casein hydrolysate formula. *J Pediatr,* 118:71-73.

Schwartz, RH, Amonette, MS (1991). Cow milk protein hydrolysate infant formulas not always "hypoallergenic." *J Pediatr,* 118:839-40.

Schwartzbaum, J, et al. (1991). An exploratory study of environmental and medical factors potentially related to childhood cancer. *Med Pediatr Oncol,* 19(2):115-21.

Scott-Emuakpor, MM, Okafor, UA (1986). Comparative study of morbidity and mortality of breastfed and bottle fed Nigerian infants. *East African Med J,* 63:452-57.

Seward, JF, Sercula, MK (1984). Infant feeding and growth. *Pediatrics,* 74 (4, pt 2):728-62.

Shahid, NS, Sack, DA, Rahman, M, Alan, AN, Rahman, N (1988). Risk factors for persistent diarrhea. *Br Med J,* 297:1036-38.

Shepherd, NF, Walker, WA (1988). The role of breastmilk in the development of the gastrointestinal tract. *Nutr Rev,* 46:1-8.

Siimes, MA, Vuori, E, Kuitunen, P (1979). Breastmilk iron—a declining concentration during the course of lactation. *Acta Paediatr Scand*, 68:29-31.

Smith, HW, Crabb, WE (1961). The faecal bacterial flora of animals and man: Its development in the young. *J Pathol Bacteril*, 82:53-66.

Spika, JS, Shaffer, N, Hargrett-Bean, N, Collin, S, MacDonald, KL, Blake, PA (1989). Risk factors for infant botulism in the United States. *Am J Dis Child*, 143:828-32.

Stephens, S, Dolby, JM, Montreuil, J, Spik, G (1980). Differences in inhibition of the growth of commensal and enteropathogenic strains of *Escherichia coli* by lactotransferrin and secretory immunoglobulin A isolated from human milk. *Immunology*, 41:597-603.

Takala, AK, Eskola, J, Palmgren, J, Ronnberg, PR, Kela, E, Rekola, P, Makela, PH (1989). Risk factors of invasive *Haemophilus influenzae* Type B disease among children in Finland. *J Pediatr*, 115:694-701.

Taylor, B, Wadsworth, J (1984). Breastfeeding and child development at five years of age. *Dev Med Child Neurol*, 26:73-80.

Temboury, MC, Otero, A, Polanco, I, Arribas, E (1994). Influence of breast-feeding on the infant's intellectual development. *J Pediatr Gastroenterol Nutr*, 18:32-36.

Tupasi, TE, Velmonte, MA, Sanvictores, MEG, Abraham, L, De Leon, LE, Tan, SA, Miguel, CA, Saniel, MC (1988). Determinants of morbidity and mortality due to acute respiratory infections: Implication for intervention. *J Infect Dis*, 157:615-23.

Uauy, RD, Birch, DG, Birch, EE, et al. (1990). Effect of dietary omega-3 fatty acids on retinal function of very-low-birthweight neonates. *Pediatr Res*, 28:485-92.

Uauy, RD, Birch, EE, Birch, DG, et al. (1992). Visual and brain function measurements in studies of n-3 fatty acid requirements of infants. *J Pediatr*, 120:S168-80.

Uraizee, F, Gross, SJ (1989). Improved feeding tolerance and reduced incidence of sepsis in sick, very low birthweight (VLBW) infants fed maternal milk. *Pediatr Res*, 25:298A.

Victoria, CG, Smith, PG, Vaughan, JP, Nobre, LC, Lombardi, C, Teixeira, AM, Fuchs, SC, Moreira, LB, Gigante, LP, Barros, FC (1989). Infant feeding and deaths to diarrhea: A case-control study. *Amer J Epidemiol*, 120(5):1032-41.

Villalpando, S, De Santiago, S (1990). Breastfeeding and protein metabolism [Spanish]. *Boletin Medico del Hospital Infantil de Mexico*, 47(3):181-85.

Walker, M (1993). A fresh look at the risk of artificial infant feeding. *J Hum Lact*, 9(2):97-107.

Weisz-Carrington, P, Roux, ME, McWilliams, M, Phillips-Quagliata, JM, Lamm, ME (1978). Hormonal induction of the secretory immune system in the mammary gland. *Proc Natl Acad Sci USA*, 75:2928-32.

Welliver, RC, Wong, DT, Sun, M, McCarty, N (1986). Parainfluenza virus bronchiolitis. *Am J Dis Child*, 140:34-40

Whitehead, RG, Paul, AA (1984). Growth charts and the assessment of infant feeding practices in the Western world and in developing countries. *Early Hum Dev*, 9: 187-207.

Whittle, BJR, Esplugues, JV (1989) PAF. In: Barnes, PJ, Page, CP, Henson, PM (Eds), *Platelet-Activating Factor and Human Disease* (pp. 198-219). Blackwell Scientific Publishers: Oxford.

Widdowson, EM, Dickerson, JWT (1964). Chemical composition of the body. In: Comar, CL, Bronner, F (Eds), *Mineral Metabolism, An Advanced Treatise*, Vol. II, Part A (pp. 1-247). Academic Press: New York

World Health Organization (WHO) (1985). *Energy and Protein Requirements*. Report of a joint FAO/WHO/UNO meeting, Geneva. *WHO Tech Rep Ser*, 724:84-89.

Wright, A (1985). Atopic dermatits and essential fatty acids: A biochemical basis for atopy? *Acta Dermato Venereol*, 114(suppl):143-45.

Wright, A, et al. (1989). Breastfeeding and lower-respiratory-tract illness in the first year of life. *Br Med J*, 299:946-49.

Wright, S, Bolton, C (1989). Breastmilk fatty acids in mothers of children with atopic exzema. *Br J Nutr*, 62:693-97.

Yang, CP, Weiss, NS, Band PR, Gallagher, RP, White, E, Daling, JR (1993). History of lactation and breast cancer risk. *Amer J Epidemiol*, 138(12):1050-56.

ADDITIONAL READINGS

Carlson, SE (1989). Polyunsaturated fatty acids and infant nutrition. In: Galli, C, Simopoulos, AP, (Eds), *Dietary Omega-3 and Omega-6 Fatty Acids: Biological Effects and Nutritional Essentiality* (pp. 147-58). Plenum Press: New York.

Carver, JD, Pimental, B, Cox, WI, et al. (1991). Dietary nucleotide effects upon immune function in infants. *Pediatrics*, 88:359-63.

Chen, Y (1989). Synergistic effect of passive smoking and artificial feeding on hospitalization for respiratory illness in early childhood. *Chest*, 95:1004-7.

Clark, K, Makrides, M, Neumann, M, et al. (1992). Determination of the optimal ratio of lineleic to alphalinolenic acid in infant formulas. *J Pediatr*, 120:S151-58.

Dumas, K, Pakter, J, Krongard, E, et al. (1988). Postnatal medical and epidemiological risk factors for the sudden infant death syndrome. In: Harper, RM, Hoffman, JH (Eds), *Sudden Infant Death Syndrome: Risk Factors and Basic Mechanisms* (pp. 187-201). PMA Publishing Corp: New York.

Farquharson, J, Cockburn, F, Patrick, WA, et al. (1992). Infant cerebral cortex phospholipid fatty-acid composition and diet. *Lancet*, 340(8823):810-13.

Finberg, L (1986). Too little water has become too much: The changing epidemilogy of water balance and convulsions in infant diarrhea. *Am J Dis Child*, 140:521.

Freundlich, M, Zilleruelo, G, Abitbol, C, et al. (1985). Infant formula as a cause of aluminum toxicity in neonatal uraemia. *Lancet*, 2(8454):527-29.

Gardner, L (1986). Neonatal tetany and high phosphate infant formulas. *Am J Dis Child*, 140:853-54.

Gerbra, JJ, Gearhart, PJ, Kamat, R, Robertson, SM, Tseng, J (1976). Origin and differentiation of lymphocytes involved in the secretory IgA response. *Quant Biol,* 41: 201-15.

Goldman, AS, Atkinson, SA, Hanson, LA (Eds) (1987). *Human Lactation 3: The Effects of Human Milk on the Recipient Infants* (pp. 251-59). Plenum Press: New York.

Goldman, AS, Goldblum, RM (1990). Human milk: Immunologic-nutritional relationships. *Ann NY Acad Sci,* 587:236-45.

Goldman, AS, Ham Pong, AJ, Goldblum, RM (1985). Host defenses: Development and maternal contributions. *Adv Pediatr,* 32:71-100.

Greco, L, Auricchio, S, Mayer, M, et al. (1988). Case-control study on nutrition risk factors in celiac disease. *J Pediatr Gastroenterol Nutr,* 7:395-99.

Grossman, H, Duggan, E, McCamman, A, et al. (1990). The dietary chloride deficiency syndrome. *Pediatrics,* 86:366-74.

Hamosh, M (1987). Lipid metabolism in premature infants. *Biol Neonate,* 52(suppl 1):50-64.

Hamosh, M, Bitman, J (1992). Human milk in disease: Lipid composition. *Lipids,* 27:848-57.

Hamosh, M., Goldman, AS (Eds) (1986). *Human Lactation 2: Maternal and Environmental Factors* (pp. 581-88). Plenum Press: New York.

Host, A, Husby, S, Osterballe, O (1988). A prospective study of cow's milk allergy in exclusively breastfed infants. *Acta Paediatr Scand,* 77:663-70.

Howell, RR, Morriss, FH, Pickering, LK (1986). *Human Milk in Infant Nutrition and Health.* Charles C Thomas: Springfield, MO.

Jatsyk, GV, Kuvaeva, IB, Gribakin, SG (1985). Immunological protection for the neonatal gastrointestinal tract: The importance of breast feeding. *Acta Paediatr Scand,* 74:246-49.

Jeffs, SG (1989). Hazards of scoop measurements in infant feeding. *J Roy Coll Gen Pract,* 39:113.

Jensen, RG, Neville, MC (1985). *Human Lactation: Milk Components and Methodologies.* Plenum Press: New York.

Jooste P, Rossouw, L, Steenkamp, H, et al. (1991). Effects of breastfeeding on the plasma cholesterol and growth of infants. *J Pediatr Gastroenterol Nutr,* 13(3):139-42.

Kaleita, TA, Kinsbourne, M, Menkes, JH, et al. (1991). A neurobehavioral syndrome after failure to thrive on chloride-deficient formula. *Dev Med Child Neurol,* 33: 626-35.

Kallio, MJ, Salmenpera, L, Siimes, MA, et al. (1992). Exclusive breastfeeding and weaning: Effect on serum cholesterol and lipoprotein concentrations in infants during the first year of life. *Pediatrics,* 89:663-66.

Keating, JP, Schears, GJ, Dodge, PR (1991). Oral water intoxication in infants, an American epidemic. *Am J Dis Child,* 145:985-90.

Koo, WWK, Kaplan, LA (1988). Aluminum and bone disorders with specific references to aluminum contamination of infant nutrients. *J Am Coll Nutr,* 7:199-214.

Lawrence, R (1994). *Breastfeeding: A Guide for the Medical Profession.* Mosby: St. Louis.

Lönnerdal, B, Chen, CL (1990). Effects of formula protein level and ratio on infant growth, plasma amino acids, and serum trace elements. *Acta Paediatr Scand,* 79:266-73.

Lopez, I, et al. (1990). Neutralizing activity against Herpes Simplex virus in human milk. *Breastfeeding Rev,* 11(2):56-58.

Malloy, MH, Graubard, B, Moss, H, et al. (1991). Hypochloremic metabolic alkalosis from ingestion of a chloride-deficient infant formula: Outcome 9 and 10 years later. *Pediatrics,* 87:811-22.

Manku, MS, Horrobin, DF, Morse, N, Kyte, N, Kyte, V, Jenkins, K, Wright, S, Burton, JL (1982). Reduced levels of prostaglandin precursors in the blood of atopic patients: Defective delta-6-desaturase function as a biochemical basis for atopy. *Prostagland Leukotr Med,* 9(6): 615-28.

May, JT (1988). Microbial contaminants and antimicrobial properties of human milk, *Microbiol Sci,* 5:42-46.

McJunkin, JE, Bithoney, WG, McCormick, MC (1987). Errors in formula concentration in an outpatient population. *J Pediatr,* 111:848-50.

McTiernan, A, Thomas, DB (1986). Evidence for a protective effect of lactation on risk of breast cancer in young women—Results from a case-control study. *Am J Epidemiol,* 124:353-58.

Merrett, TG, Burr, ML, Butland, BK, et al. (1988). Infant feeding and allergy: Twelve-month prospective study of 500 babies born in allergic families. *Ann Allergy,* 61(6, pt 2):13-20.

Money, DFL (1978). Feeding and the sudden infant death syndrome: Classification of 224 New Zealand cases by the milk food given. *NZ J Med Sci,* 21:547-51.

Muytjens, HL, Roelofs-Willomse, H, Jasper, HS (1988). Quality of powdered substitutes for breastmilk with regard to members of the family Enterobacteriaceae. *J Clin Microbiol,* 26:743-46.

Patton, S, Houston, GE (1987). Differences between individuals in high-MR glycoproteins form human mammary epithelial. *FEBS Lett,* 216:151-54.

Perez, A, Labbok, MH, Queenan, JT (1992). Clinical study of the lactational amenorrhoea method for family planning. *Lancet,* 339:968-70.

Quan, R, Barness, LA, Uauy, R (1990). Do infants need nucleotide supplemented formula for optimal nutrition? *J Pediatr Gastroenterol Nutr,* 11:429-34.

Rowe, B, Begg, NT, Hutchinson, DN, et al. (1987). Salmonella infections associated with consumption of infant dried milk. *Lancet,* 2(8564):900-3.

Sampson, HA, Bernhisel-Broadbent, J, Yanq, E, et al. (1991). Safety of casein hydrolysate formula in children with cow milk allergy. *J Pediatr,* 118:520-25.

Schaffer, A, Ditchek, S (1991). Current social practices leading to water intoxication in infants. *Am J Dis Child,* 145:27-28.

Simmons, BP, Gelfand, MS, Haas, M, et al. (1989). *Enterobacter sakazakii* infections in neonates associated with intrinsic contamination of a powdered infant formula. *Infect Control Hosp Epidemiol,* 10:398-401.

Simopoulos, AP (1991). Omega-3 fatty acids in health and disease and in growth and development. *Am J Clin Nutr,* 54:438-63.

Sowers, M, Corton, G, Shapiro, B, et al. (1993). Changes in bone density with lactation. *JAMA,* 269:3130-35.

Sullivan, P (1989). Canada's infant-death rate lowest in Americas, but situation elsewhere tragic. *Can Med Assoc J,* 140:324.

United Kingdom National Case-Control Study Group (1993). Breast-feeding and risk of breast cancer in young women. *Br Med J,* 307:17-20.

Whorwell, PJ, Holdstock, G, Whorwell, GM, et al. (1979). Bottlefeeding, early gastroenteritis, and inflammatory bowel disease. *Br Med J,* (6160):382.

Willoughby, A, Braubard, BI, Hocker, A, et al. (1990). Population-based study of the developmental outcome of children exposed to chloride-deficient infant formula. *Pediatrics,* 85:485-90.

Willoughby, A, Moss, HA, Hubbard, VS, et al. (1987). Developmental outcome in children exposed to chloride-deficient formula. *Pediatrics,* 79:851-57.

Yoo, KY, Tajima K, Kuroishi, T, Hirose, K, Yoshida, M, Miura, S, Murai, H (1992). Independent protective effect of lactation against breast cancer: A case-control study in Japan. *Amer J Epidemiol,* 135(7):726-33.

Zeigler, E, Fomon, S (1989). Potential renal solute load of infant formulas. *J Nutr,* 119:1785-88.

CHAPTER 3

Breastfeeding Support Policies and Resources

SECTION A

The Promotion of Breastfeeding with Supportive Policies

Jan Simpson, RN, BSN, IBCLC
Rebecca F. Black, MS, RD/LD, IBCLC

LEARNING OBJECTIVES

At the completion of this section, the learner will be able to do the following:

1. State how the health-care professional's attitude, routines, and verbal and nonverbal responses influence a mother's decision to breastfeed and her success.
2. Discuss the national breastfeeding objective adopted by the U.S. Surgeon General at the 1984 Surgeon General's Workshop on Breastfeeding and Human Lactation and subsequent objectives set by follow-up conferences.
3. Describe practices that discourage breastfeeding.
4. Identify strategies that will encourage and support the initiation of breastfeeding.
5. Explain how implementing the WHO/UNICEF Ten Steps to Successful Breastfeeding lays a foundation for the implementation and continuation of a successful breastfeeding experience.

OUTLINE

I. Global Promotion of Breastfeeding

    A. The influence of health-care professionals

    B. Surgeon General's Workshop on Breastfeeding and Human Lactation

    C. WHO International Code of Marketing of Breastmilk Substitutes

D. Innocenti Declaration

E. World Declartation and Plan of Action for Nutrition

II. Promotion of Breastfeeding in the Health-Care Environment

A. Ten Steps to Successful Breastfeeding

B. U.S. Breastfeeding Health Initiative

C. Establishment and implementation of state and community coalitions

---

PRE-TEST

For questions 1 to 10, choose the single best answer from the following key (do the comments or actions encourage or discourage breastfeeding):

A. Encourage   B. Discourage

1. Infant is put to breast immediately in delivery room.

2. Television in clinic showing nonsponsored breastfeeding educational videos.

3. Schedule feedings despite breastfeeding mother's wishes.

4. Pictures of women bottle feeding displayed in clinic and hospital.

5. Rooming-in of mother and infant.

6. Mother and infant are separated at birth.

7. Breastfeeding mother told she "is not doing it right" and is interrupted and corrected despite her efforts.

8. Breastfeeding mother given formula gift pack on her hospital discharge.

9. Woman sees others breastfeeding.

10. Staff initiates discussion regarding woman's intention to breastfeed during the prenatal and postpartum periods.

For questions 11 to 17, choose the single best answer.

11. The beginning of any successful breastfeeding program involves obtaining support and commitment from:

    A. administration.

    B. doctors and nurses.

    C. nutrition specialist.

    D. counselors.

    E. All of the above

12. The continued breastfeeding education of all staff coming into contact with women and infants is imperative for the following reason(s):

    A. It promotes correct and consistent breastfeeding advice and instructions being given out by all staff.

    B. It ensures that breastfeeding knowledge of staff is up-to-date with correct and current breastfeeding information.

   C. Continued education in the area of breastfeeding is not a necessary component for staff coming into contact with women and infants.
   D. Both A and B

13. Breastfeeding information should be made readily accessible to all women during:

   A. postpartum period.
   B. Both A and C
   C. prenatal period.
   D. None of the above

14. Following birth, breastfeeding mothers should be assisted in putting their infants to the breast:

   A. Immediately following delivery (unless medically contraindicated).
   B. After the infant has been sent to the nursery for an assessment and bath.
   C. After the mother has rested or had a good night's sleep.
   D. Both B and C

15. If the breastfeeding relationship must be interrupted, instructions to the mother should include which of the following:

   A. Methods of breastmilk expression appropriate to her situation
   B. Storage of expressed breastmilk
   C. Milk expression is not necessary when breastfeedings are missed. The mother should just wait until the infant is able to be put back to breast.
   D. Both A and B

16. Giving breastfed infants water following a nursing session is necessary because:

   A. it is required in order to maintain water homeostasis.
   B. there is no water content in breastmilk.
   C. it can prevent hyperbilirubinemia.
   D. water supplements are not needed. None of the above is true.

17. On-demand breastfeeding:

   A. fosters positive breastfeeding relationships, decreasing problems such as engorgement.
   B. establishes adequate milk production.
   C. promotes decreased bilirubin levels and infant weight gain.
   D. All of the above

For questions 18 to 20, choose the best answer from the following key:
   A. True   **B. False**

18. Policies allowing complementary or supplementary feeds to breastfeeding infants should be avoided unless medically indicated.

19. Inconsistencies in breastfeeding instruction and information given out by health-care workers discourages breastfeeding success.

20. All pregnant women should be informed of the benefits of breastfeeding.

Global Promotion of Breastfeeding

Breastmilk's superiority over any substitute has been established for nutritional, biochemical, anti-infective, psychological, economic, and contraceptive reasons. Health-care providers should consider the promotion and support of breastfeeding a priority of the highest order. Educating expectant mothers in the perinatal period, as well as in the prenatal period, combined with a hospital routine supportive of the breastfeeding relationship, has been established to increase breastfeeding incidence and duration (Winikoff & Baer, 1980).

THE INFLUENCE OF HEALTH-CARE PROFESSIONALS

It is a goal that health-care settings, whether hospitals, physicians' offices, health departments, or clinics, project a positive and supportive breastfeeding environment and promote it as the finest form of infant nutrition. This can be done by implementing policies and procedures that are pro-breastfeeding. Many times when this type of environment is not found, it is because of a lack of breastfeeding education or outdated information still in practice by health-care professionals. This not only shows a need for educating new health-care professionals as to the many aspects of the lactating mother and child, but the need to provide continuing breastfeeding education consisting of current information to all members of the health-care team who may come into contact with the breastfeeding family. Education of the health-care staff coming into contact with the mother or infant is essential for the success of a breastfeeding promotion program (Best, 1991).

Figure 3A–1

Supportive nursing care for breastfeeding mother and baby.

Source: From Woessner, C, Lauwers, J, Bernard, B (1991). *Breastfeeding Today. A Mother's Companion*, p. 60. Avery Publishing Co: Garden City, NY. Reprinted with permission.

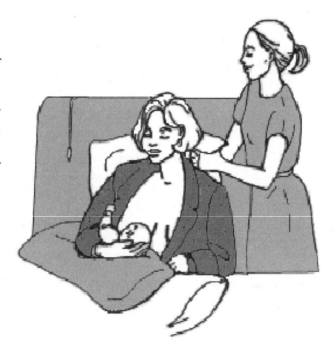

Health-care professionals wield a strong influence on infant-feeding practices by their attitudes, routines, and verbal and nonverbal support (Kearney, 1988; Reiff & Essock-Vitale, 1985). They are able to help provide conditions in which the breastfeeding relationship can thrive and grow or fail.

SURGEON GENERAL'S WORKSHOP ON BREASTFEEDING AND HUMAN LACTATION

Many of our nation's top health-care professionals gathered on June 11 and 12, 1984, in Rochester, New York, for the Surgeon General's Workshop on Breastfeeding and Human Lactation. This workshop resulted from a goal set by the World Health Organization (WHO) in 1978: "Health for All by the Year 2000." The United States had earlier set a series of objectives and goals to be achieved by 1990. One of the "Health Promotion/Disease Prevention Objectives for the Nation" was addressed at the workshop and was presented by the Surgeon General C. Everett Koop, MD, ScD. This objective was that by the year 1990: "The proportion of women who breastfeed their babies at hospital discharge should be increased to 75%, and the percentage of those still breastfeeding at 6 months of age should be increased to 35%." When the national goal was adopted in 1978, statistics showed the proportion of mothers and infants breastfeeding at hospital discharge at 45%, and 21% continuing breastfeeding at 6 months of age (U.S. Department of Health and Human Services, 1984). In 1988, 54% were breastfeeding at discharge and 21% were breastfeeding at 5 to 6 months of age. The goals were not met by 1990 and were again affirmed as goals for the year 2000 with the desired duration at 6 months increased to 50% (USDHHS, 1991).

Along with the discussion of this national objective, six recommendations with proposed approaches to aid in the progress of achieving this national objective were introduced. The recommendations as stated in the Followup Report are as follows (USDHHS, 1985):

- Improve professional education in human lactation and breastfeeding.
- Develop public education and promotional efforts.
- Strengthen the support for breastfeeding in the health-care system.
- Develop a broad range of support services in the community.
- Initiate a national breastfeeding promotion effort directed toward employed women.
- Expand research on human lactation and breastfeeding.

Endeavors to increase breastfeeding incidence and duration in our nation had occurred in many areas even prior to the Surgeon General's workshop. Following the workshop, however, many new efforts were initiated, and many prior efforts broadened in response to its recommendations and objectives.

Since the 1984 Surgeon General's Workshop, three publications have been developed to provide updates on the promotion of breastfeeding. The following resources for breastfeeding information are considered invaluable and inspirational:

- The Report of the Surgeon General's Workshop on Breastfeeding and Human Lactation (1984)

- Followup Report: Surgeon General's Workshop on Breastfeeding and Human Lactation (1985)
- Second Followup Report: Surgeon General's Workshop on Breastfeeding and Human Lactation (1991)

WHO INTERNATIONAL CODE OF MARKETING OF BREASTMILK SUBSTITUTES

On May 21, 1981, the WHO International Code of Marketing of Breastmilk Substitutes was approved by a vote of 118 to 1 (the United States cast the only opposing vote) by the World Health Assembly. The code was developed with the intention that it was to be adopted by governments to protect the health of infants by preventing inappropriate marketing of breastmilk substitutes (IBFAN/IOCU, 1990). The code sets minimal standards to assist with the promotion of breastfeeding as the superior form of infant nutrition. The code does not seek to ban the sale of formula or prevent educating the medical community about products (see Table 3A–1).

WHO and UNICEF published a joint statement in 1989 entitled *Protecting, Promoting, and Supporting Breast-Feeding: The Special Role of Maternity Services.* The statement made recommendations for educating and supporting lactating mothers and the role health services should play in the promotion of breastfeeding. In 1994, the WHO reaffirmed the code. The United States voted in favor of the code, reversing its position taken in 1981.

On August 1, 1990, at a WHO/UNICEF meeting, "Breastfeeding in the 90s: A Global Initiative," the Innocenti Declaration was adopted. This declaration was developed and adopted by high-level policymakers from 32 governments and United Nations' agencies. Four goals were set to be met by 1995 (IBFAN/IOCU, 1990):

1. The establishment of National Breastfeeding Coordinators.
2. The practice of Ten Steps to Successful Breastfeeding by maternity services.
3. The implementation of the WHO code.

Table 3A–1 WHO Code for Marketing Breastmilk Substitutes

- No advertising of these products to the public.
- Information to health workers should be scientific and factual.
- No free samples to mothers.
- All information on artificial feeding, including the labels, should explain the benefits of breastfeeding, and the costs and hazards associated with artificial feeding.
- No promotion of products in health-care facilities.
- Unsuitable products, such as condensed milk, should not be promoted for babies.
- No company mothercraft nurses to advise mothers.
- All products should be of a high quality and take into account the climatic and storage conditions of the country where they are used.
- No gifts or personal samples to health workers.
- No words or pictures idealizing artificial feeding, including pictures of infants on the products.

Source: IBFAN/IOCU (1990). *Protecting Infant Health—A Health Worker's Guide to the International Code of Marketing of Breastmilk Substitutes*, 6th ed. IBFAN/IOCU: Penang, Malaysia. Reprinted with permission.

4. Enactment of enforceable laws for protecting the breastfeeding rights of employed women.

INNOCENTI DECLARATION*

Recognizing that breastfeeding is a unique process, being a single activity that:

- Lowers infant mortality and morbidity primarily by lowering incidence and severity of infectious illnesses
- Provides high-quality nutrition for infants and contributes to their growth and development
- Contributes to women's health by reducing risks of certain cancers and anemia and by increasing the spacing between pregnancies
- Provides economic benefits to the family and the nation
- When successfully carried out, provides most women with a sense of satisfaction

Recent research has found that these benefits increase with increased exclusivity of breastfeeding in infancy and increased duration of breastfeeding with complementary foods, and program interventions can result in positive changes in breastfeeding behavior.

WE THEREFORE DECLARE that, for optimal maternal and child health and nutrition, all women should be enabled to practice exclusive breastfeeding and all infants should be fed exclusively on breastmilk from birth for the first 4 to 6 months of life. Children should continue to be breastfed, while receiving appropriate and adequate complementary foods, for up to 2 years of age or beyond. This child-feeding ideal is to be achieved by creating an environment of awareness and support so that women can breastfeed in this manner.

Measures should be taken to ensure that women are adequately nourished for the optimal health of themselves and their families. Furthermore, ensuring that all women also have access to family planning information and services allows them to sustain breastfeeding and avoid shortened birth intervals that may compromise their health and nutritional status and that of their children.

Attainment of the goal demands, in many countries, reinforcement of a breastfeeding culture and vigorously defending it against incursions of a bottle-feeding culture. This requires commitment and advocacy for social mobilization, utilizing to the fullest the prestige and authority of acknowledged leaders of society in all walks of life.

Efforts must be made to increase the confidence of women in their ability to breastfeed. Such empowerment involves the removal of constraints and influences that manipulate women's perceptions and behavior, often by subtle and indirect means. This requires sensitivity, continued vigilance, and a responsive and comprehensive communications strategy involving all media addressing all levels of society.

All countries should develop national breastfeeding policies and set national targets (impact and process) for the 1990s. They should establish a national system for monitoring the attainment of the targets, and develop indicators such as the

---

*This section is adapted from *On the Protection, Promotion, and Support of Breastfeeding* (August 1, 1990; Florence, Italy).

prevalence of exclusive breastfeeding at discharge from maternity hospital and the prevalence of exclusive breastfeeding at the age of four months.

National authorities are further urged to integrate their breastfeeding policies into their overall health and development policies, seeing to it that they are not in conflict. In doing so, they should reinforce all the actions that complement breastfeeding programs such as safe motherhood, prevention and treatment of common childhood diseases, and family planning.

Possible Operational Targets

By the year 1995, all countries should have:

- Appointed a National Breastfeeding Coordinator of appropriate authority, and established a National Breastfeeding Committee with membership from relevant government departments and nongovernment organizations;
- Ensured that every maternity facility fully practices all of the "Ten Steps to Successful Breastfeeding" (see page 150);
- Given effect to the International Code of Marketing of Breastmilk Substitutes and subsequent relevant World Health Assembly resolutions in their entirety;
- Enacted imaginative legislation protecting the breastfeeding rights of working women and established means for its enforcement.

We call on international organizations:

- to encourage and support national authorities in their own planning and implementation of national breastfeeding policies;
- to support national surveys and the setting up of national goals and targets for action;
- to draw up their own action strategies for protection, promotion, and support of breastfeeding, including global monitoring and evaluation.

Figure 3A–2
Woman Breastfeeding Toddler.
Source: UNICEF, *Tomemos la iniciativa en pro de los ninos!* p. 11. Reprinted with permission.

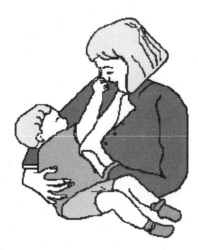

WORLD DECLARATION AND PLAN OF ACTION FOR NUTRITION

Responding to the urging for governmental planning in breastfeeding and other nutrition issues, 1,300 delegates from 159 nations came together in December 1992 at the International Conference on Nutrition (ICN) to develop the World Declaration and Plan of Action for Nutrition. The 21-point World Declaration on Nutrition and accompanying Plan of Action for Nutrition is a pledge to eliminate or reduce substantially—within this decade—starvation, widespread undernutrition, and malnutrition, which constrains progress in human and societal development around the world.

The United Nations sponsored the World Summit for Children in New York during 1990 and developed the Fourth United Nations Development Decade plan. Promoting breastfeeding is one component outlined in the plan. Goals (to be reached by the year 2000) of the World Summit for Children and for the United Nations Development Decade are highlighted in Tables 3A–2 and 3A–3.

Table 3A–2   Nutrition Goals of the World Summit for Children

- Reduction in severe, as well as moderate, malnutrition among under-5 children by half of 1990 levels;
- Reduction of the rate of low birthweight (2.5 kg or less) to less than 10%;
- Reduction of iron-deficiency anemia in women by one-third of the 1990 levels;
- Virtual elimination of iodine-deficiency disorders;
- Virtual elimination of vitamin A–deficiency and its consequences, including blindness;
- Empowerment of all women to breastfeed their children exclusively for 4 to 6 months and to continue breastfeeding, with complementary food, well into the second year;
- Growth promotion and its regular monitoring to be institutionalized in all countries by the end of the 1990s;
- Dissemination of knowledge and supporting services to increase food production to ensure household food security.

Source: Adapted from report of the World Summit for Children. New York: United Nations, September 1990.

Table 3A–3   Nutrition Goals for the Fourth United Nations Development Decade

Member states must give effect to agreements already reached to make all efforts to meet four goals during the decade:

1. To eliminate starvation and death caused by famine
2. To substantially reduce malnutrition and mortality among children
3. To tangibly reduce chronic hunger
4. To eliminate major nutritional diseases

Source: Adapted from report of the World Summit for Children. New York: United Nations, September 1990.

Promotion of Breastfeeding in the Health-Care Environment

Breastfeeding is undoubtedly the healthiest and most complete form of infant nutrition available. Breastmilk's advantages far outweigh any claimed advantages of breastmilk substitutes, and its superiority has been proven in study after study. For more on breastfeeding advantages, see Chapter 2 in this module. For the sake of our children, breastfeeding must be promoted and supported in health-care environments. The clinic setting itself must show the support of breastfeeding, as well as the health-care professionals working inside. Professionals working in the field have an important role in encouraging circumstances in which the breast-feeding relationship can succeed and grow.

In support of the acceptance of breastfeeding worldwide, UNICEF and WHO have introduced a "Baby Friendly Hospital Initiative" (BFHI) campaign. The goal of this campaign is to convince health-care providers and parents around the world that breastfeeding gives babies "The Best Possible Start in Life." To achieve "baby friendly" status, a hospital must meet standards set by UNICEF and WHO in the Ten Steps to Successful Breastfeeding (see Table 3A–4). One of the goals outlined in the Innocenti Declaration signed by the United States in 1990 stated "that every facility providing maternity services fully practices all of the Ten Steps to Successful Breastfeeding set out in the 1989 joint WHO/UNICEF statement *Protecting, Promoting, and Supporting Breast-Feeding: The Special Role of Maternity Services.*

TEN STEPS TO SUCCESSFUL BREASTFEEDING

WHO/UNICEF Step #1

"Have a Written Breastfeeding Policy That Is Routinely Communicated to All Health-Care Staff."

Opinions and attitudes toward breastfeeding that are held by health-care workers may have a vital role in effecting the success or failure of a breastfeeding experience. The beginning of any successful breastfeeding program involves obtaining support and commitment from those working within the structured health-care setting. Administrative support, as well as staff support, during prenatal care, lasting throughout the postnatal-care period and beyond is essential. Health-care professionals and routines have an immense impact on infant-feeding practices decided on by the parents and the success they feel with their decision.

Correct and consistent breastfeeding advice should be offered to the breastfeeding mother. Health-care providers should have written policies to help initiate and maintain this goal. Breastfeeding policies can be written by the institution itself or by professional groups/committees. Policies will provide written guidelines and instructions that will assist all staff working with mothers and/or infants in providing the breastfeeding instruction and support needed.

Policies must be based on current breastfeeding knowledge and be supported by scientific studies and rationale. To remain up-to-date with correct information, policies must be reviewed and updated on a regular basis by knowledgeable professionals. For the policies and guidelines to work, and be carried out by all,

Table 3A–4   Ten Steps to Successful Breastfeeding

Every facility providing maternity services and care for newborn infants should:

1. Have a written breastfeeding policy that is routinely communicated to all health-care staff.
2. Train all health-care staff in skills necessary to implement this policy.
3. Inform all pregnant women about the benefits and management of breastfeeding.
4. Help mothers initiate breastfeeding within a half-hour of birth.
5. Show mothers how to breastfeed and how to maintain lactation even if they should be separated from their infants.
6. Give newborn infants no food or drink other than breastmilk, unless medically indicated.
7. Practice rooming-in. Allow mothers and infants to remain together 24 hours a day.
8. Encourage breastfeeding on demand.
9. Give no artificial teats or pacifiers (also called dummies or soothers) to breastfeeding infants.
10. Foster the establishment of breastfeeding support groups and refer mothers to them on discharge from the hospital or clinic.

Source: *Protecting, Promoting and Supporting Breast-Feeding: The Special Role of Maternity Services.* A Joint WHO/UNICEF Statement, July 1989. Reprinted with permission.

administrative personnel must see that the policies are consistently followed by those working in the area by including this as a part of the quality-indicator program and employee evaluation process. As with all aspects of health care, the care that is provided for the breastfeeding mother and infant must be evaluated to meet the high quality of care required. Public health agencies at state and local levels should publish policy statements reinforcing their commitment and support of national public health statements on breastfeeding.

WHO/UNICEF Step #2

"Train All Health-Care Staff in Skills Necessary to Implement This Policy."

After a health-care facility has administratively and actively adopted policies that protect, promote, and support the breastfeeding mother and infant, it is imperative that all employees working in the area be instructed on a regular basis to maintain an efficient level of current breastfeeding knowledge. Lactation education in-services, along with hospital breastfeeding policies, must be shared with all staff coming into contact with the mother and/or infant. When a new breastfeeding policy is implemented, staff in-services are necessary to provide a discussion of the policy and the expected outcomes. This will help facilitate comprehension and cooperation from all. Individual job or position descriptions also must emphasize individual employer expectations of employees regarding breastfeeding promotion and support.

WHO/UNICEF Step #3

"Inform All Pregnant Women about the Benefits and Management of Breastfeeding."

Breastfeeding information should be made readily accessible to all women during the prenatal period. Although many physicians acknowledge their support of breastfeeding, they do not always initiate the topic of infant feeding, and it may only be discussed if questions arise from the parents-to-be. This also seems to hold true with many other health-care professionals. Every mother has the right to make an informed choice regarding the feeding method she chooses for her child. This can only be done if the benefits and management of breastfeeding are discussed with the pregnant woman. Informed choice also means that the disadvantages or hazards of artificial feeding are reviewed with a pregnant woman. Educational programs for clients should begin in the prenatal period and continue during the hospital stay.

Although prenatal lactation education is not essential, it is optimal. Prenatally and postnatally, the client and her support person should be instructed on the physiology of lactation, infant positioning and latch-on techniques, nipple care, milk expression, and ways to avoid and manage problems, such as sore nipples or engorgement, that could be encountered while breastfeeding. Client education can be provided by one-on-one instruction, breastfeeding classes, audiovisual aids, and written materials. It is important that the materials being used to provide lactation education be evaluated on a regular basis to remain up-to-date with current breastfeeding information. The knowledge obtained by continuing research is essential for breastfeeding success.

It is extremely important to know who is producing and distributing the teaching aids and materials being provided to clients. Avoidance of formula-sponsored material under all circumstances where breastfeeding is being promoted is strongly encouraged. Reading materials and videos often supplied free of charge by formula companies may begin by providing breastfeeding information, but also may include information on artificial feeding and may emphasize breastfeeding problems. This is considered a deterrent to breastfeeding and discourages an exclusive breastfeeding relationship.

Figure 3A–3
Pregnant Woman Contemplating the Infant-Feeding Decision
Source: Ohio State University Breastfeeding Promotion Project, 1986. Reprinted with permission.

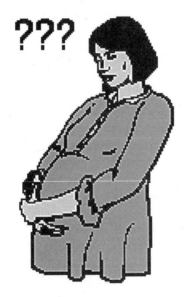

Prenatal assessment of the pregnant woman's breasts and nipples may assist in the detection of possible difficulties that may be encountered when breastfeeding begins. Nipple preparation by rough manipulation, such as buffing with towels, has been shown not to prevent sore nipples and is no longer advocated. The abandonment of nipple preparation does not negate the idea of a woman touching her breasts to become comfortable with handling them prior to her baby's birth. If during the prenatal assessment, it is noted that the pregnant woman has flat or inverted nipples, the need for treatment should be identified and initiated in the last trimester to help prevent problems from occurring when breastfeeding is started (see Module 2, *The Process of Breastfeeding*, Chapter 1).

WHO/UNICEF Step #4

"Help Mothers Initiate Breastfeeding within a Half-Hour after Birth."

Mothers should be assisted in putting their infants to the breast as soon as possible, immediately following delivery, to take advantage of the infant's strong sucking reflex that occurs during the first 1 to 2 hours of life. The sucking reflex is at its strongest peak during the first 30 minutes following birth. Postponing the gratification of this sucking reflex may cause the infant to have problems learning to suck properly at the breast at a later point in time. Maintaining this mother–infant contact immediately following birth not only aids in the maternal bonding process, but assists in encouraging a positive breastfeeding relationship and establishing a sense of self-confidence in the new mother. It has been shown that women who initiated early breastfeedings with prolonged contact tended to breastfeed for a longer duration (Winikoff et al., 1987; Winikoff & Baer, 1980; Woolridge et al., 1985).

There are many physical attributes to immediate nursing after delivery. For the infant, body temperature is maintained by skin-to-skin contact with mother. The ingestion of colostrum provides immunologic advantages and acts as a laxative, aiding in the expulsion of the meconium, thus decreasing the incidence of excessive hyperbilirubinemia (DeCarvalho et al., 1982; Ostler, 1979). Evidence suggests that the skin-to-skin contact immediately following delivery strengthens the mother-to-infant bond, creating a greater chance of prolonged breastfeeding. Klaus and Kennell (1976) reported that 45 minutes of contact following birth was related to a greater duration of breastfeeding. For the mother, the stimulation of breastfeeding results in the release of the hormone oxytocin, which causes the uterus to contract and aids in the inhibition of excessive vaginal bleeding, as well as aiding in the return of the uterus to its prepregnancy state. Engorgement of the breast or breasts is reduced or prevented by early and frequent removal of milk from the breast.

If birth complications occur, immediate breastfeeding of the infant following delivery may be contraindicated. Examples of situations in which this may apply include:

- An infant's Apgar score is less than 6 at 5 minutes.
- An infant is having respiratory distress.
- An infant is premature—less than 36 weeks gestation
- A mother is heavily sedated

In these extreme cases, the mother should be offered immediate support and encouragement and be allowed to begin the breastfeeding relationship as soon as possible. Those mothers who must be separated from their infants for medical reasons should be instructed on milk expression and how to start storage (see Module 2, *The Process of Breastfeeding*, Chapter 3).

WHO/UNICEF Step #5

"Show Mothers How to Breastfeed, and How to Maintain Lactation Even If They Should Be Separated from Their Infants."

All mothers who are breastfeeding, or planning to breastfeed their infants, should be educated on the lactation process, including positioning, latching-on techniques, on-demand feeding, milk-intake assessment, nipple care, and other time-appropriate skills and techniques (see Module 2, *The Process of Breastfeeding*, Chapter 1). By initiating early education, many of the problems that can be associated with breastfeeding may be avoided. Frequent evaluation of the lactation process, especially during the early part of the breastfeeding relationship, can assist in the identification of areas that may require additional support.

If the breastfeeding relationship must be interrupted, the mother should be instructed on ways to express and store her milk to maintain lactation for when her infant is able to be put to her breasts. These mothers may require additional emotional encouragement and support.

WHO/UNICEF Step #6

"Give Newborn Infants No Food or Drink Other Than Breastmilk, Unless Medically Indicated."

Giving the breastfeeding infant supplements (replacement feeds) or complements (additional feeds of breastmilk substitutes) has been shown to be a contributing factor to a failed breastfeeding relationship by various lactation research studies. Not only may it cause nipple confusion when given by an artificial teat, but the infant who receives the supplement or complement feed becomes full and will go longer intervals between feedings, or may take less from the breast at the next feeding because of fullness. The breasts may become engorged from the missed feedings or the inadequate emptying, and this can eventually lead to diminished milk production (AAP/CPS, 1978; AAP, 1985; AAP/ACOG, 1988).

Infants who are being exclusively fed from the breasts do not require water supplementation to maintain water homeostasis (Sachdev, 1991). The new mother must be encouraged that her breastmilk alone is enough to provide complete nourishment and adequate hydration for her newborn infant. Water supplements have not been proven to prevent or cure infants from becoming jaundiced and provide infants with a substance of no caloric value. If a mother feels her infant "needs more," encourage frequent, longer nursing sessions (Brown et al., 1986; DeCarvalho et al., 1982).

The routine distribution of free gift packs provided by formula companies is strongly discouraged because it may give the new mother an unspoken message that her breastmilk alone is not enough to satisfy her infant's nourishment needs. The distribution of artificial breastmilk samples have been reported to be associated with a higher incidence of bottle feeding at one month and the introduction of solids at two months of age (Bergevin et al., 1983). These gift packs should not be given to a breastfeeding mother unless requested by the mother or ordered by the physician.

WHO/UNICEF Step #7

"Practice Rooming-In—Allow Mothers and Infants to Remain Together 24 Hours a Day."

Rooming-in, allowing the mother and infant to remain together, has numerous benefits for the breastfeeding relationship. It provides the new mother with the opportunity to breastfeed her infant on-demand, whether it be maternal or infant demand, while observing for early hunger cues. Mother–infant rooming-in fosters a positive breastfeeding environment and promotes breastfeeding success and maternal confidence.

WHO/UNICEF Step #8

"Encourage Breastfeeding on Demand."

Breastmilk is easily digested, usually within one to one-and-a-half hours after ingestion. This is much faster than breastmilk substitutes, so a breastfed infant may require frequent feedings. On-demand feedings not only foster positive breastfeeding relationships between mothers and infants, but establish adequate milk production, infant weight gain, decreased bilirubin levels, and a decrease in engorgement.

WHO/UNICEF Step #9

"Give No Artificial Teats or Pacifiers (Also Called Dummies or Soothers) to Breastfeeding Infants."

Sucking from an artificial teat requires a different tongue movement than does the infant sucking from the breast. Thus, the breastfed infant who is given an artificial teat may develop the problem of nipple confusion, and the effectiveness of breast-feeding is decreased. Encourage the new mother to exclusively breastfeed her infant during the early weeks of life to assist in the avoidance of such a problem. If feeding at the breast must be interrupted, or supplements or complements are medically in-dicated, encourage an alternative to the artificial teat for introducing the feeds (dropper, spoon, cup, finger feeding, periodontal syringe, nursing supplementer).

The overuse of pacifiers may contribute to multiple problems. The suck is differ-ent, possibly causing an ineffective suckle at the breast or rejection of the breast. The infant may have his or her sucking needs met by the pacifier; this may lead to decreased time at the breast or a decreased milk supply, which can result in prob-lems such as engorgement and slow weight gain. Putting the infant to the breast for more frequent breastfeeding rather than excessively using the pacifier is rec-ommended (see Figure 3A–4).

Discharge gift packs containing bottles, artificial teats in the forms of bottle nip-ples and pacifiers, and formula that the mother may receive when leaving the hos-pital are deterrents to a successful and lasting breastfeeding relationship. Gift packs should not be given to the breastfeeding couple unless specifically re-quested by the family or ordered by the physician. The distribution of free for-mula gift packs has been associated with shortened duration of breastfeeding in many cases. Health-care providers may want to consider the option of developing free gift packs designed especially for the breastfeeding mother that would pro-mote the continuity of a successful and satisfying breastfeeding relationship.

Figure 3A–4

Breastfeeding Promotion Slogan

Source: Breastfeeding Promotion Project. Registered trademark of *Global Graffiti.* Reprinted with permission.

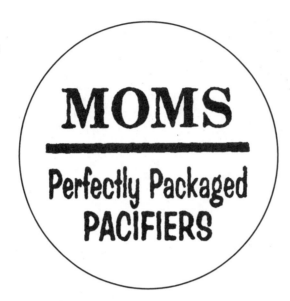

WHO/UNICEF Step #10

"Foster the Establishment of Breastfeeding Support Groups and Refer Mothers to Them on Discharge from the Hospital or Clinic."

Breastfeeding support groups (Figure 3A–5) are of vital importance as they provide lactation education, guidance, and breastfeeding assistance beyond hospital discharge as well as prenatally. The continuity of breastfeeding support following the birth of the infant is imperative in many situations and valued in all.

Hospital, clinic, and community support are significant contributors to a successful breastfeeding experience. It is ideal if breastfeeding education can begin in the prenatal period, with prenatal breastfeeding classes and/or breastfeeding support groups, combined with physician encouragement and support. During the hospital stay, lactation education continues and builds on what was learned during the prenatal period. It is imperative that all hospital/clinic staff continue to provide current and consistent breastfeeding information, support, and encouragement. Many lactation consultants and WIC programs provide postpartum services for breastfeeding families.

U.S. BREASTFEEDING HEALTH INITIATIVE

The national Healthy Mothers, Healthy Babies (HMHB) coalition completed an 18-month feasibility study of WHO/UNICEF'S Baby Friendly Hospital Initiative (BFHI) in 1994. The study was sponsored through the Maternal and Child Health Bureau of the U.S. Department of Health and Human Services.

To complete the feasibility study, an expert work group (EWG) of organizational designees was convened. Staff/consultant expertise reviewed relevant literature,

Figure 3A–5

Breastfeeding Support Group.

Source: The Population Council (1989). *A Mother's Guide to Breastfeeding*, p.3. Reprinted with permission.

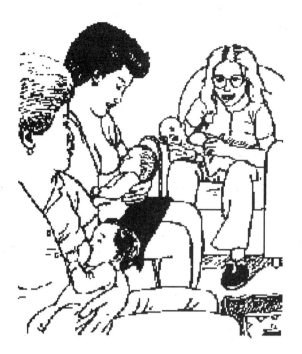

conducted the necessary information gathering and analysis and tested credentialing approaches. The study was charged with doing the following:

1. Determine the appropriateness of the 10 criteria of the BFHI for the United States and recommend adaptations if needed.
2. Inform organizations that will review and ratify the initiative with the group's consensus on the hospital criteria;
3. Discuss and recommend how the hospital-certification process of BFHI should be handled and propose approaches for a feasibility testing;
4. Consider literature review, procedural testing, hospital interests, and legal ramifications for a voluntary, private-sector BFHI.

The EWG members reached consensus on the following recommendations (HMHB, 1994):

1. Adapt the UNICEF/WHO Baby Friendly Hospital Initiative for the United States by revising the Ten Steps and Global Criteria as recommended by the EWG.
2. Name the initiative in the United States the "U.S. Breastfeeding Health Initiative" (U.S. BfHI).
3. Establish a privately supported, national, independent review body to implement the initiative and to determine the requirements for hospital recognition.
4. Develop a self-assessment process based on the continuous quality improvement concept.
5. Make the national review body the implementing agency for the U.S. BfHI recognition program.

6. Secure a trademark for "U.S. Breastfeeding Health Initiative."
7. Make implementation of the U.S. BFHI independent of any follow-up by the U.S. federal government with UNICEF.

Ten Steps and Criteria for the U.S. BFHI

Step One

Maintain an written breastfeeding policy that is communicated to all health-care staff.

- Breastmilk is the standard for infant feeding.
- The hospital will have a written policy that addresses the implementation of all Ten Steps and encourages breastfeeding.*
- The hospital will identify the health-care professional within the health-care facility who will have responsibility for the development, update, evaluation, revision, and communication of the hospital policy with the other staff who take care of mothers and infants. The designated health-care professional will ensure that the policy is available to all pertinent staff and that it is communicated to all new employees during their orientation and at other times as determined by the health-care facility.
- The hospitals will prominently display the Ten Steps in all areas of the health-care facility that serve mothers, infants, and/or children, including labor and delivery, the postpartum unit, all infant-care areas, affiliated prenatal-care areas, and the emergency room.

Step Two

- Train all pertinent health-care staff in skills necessary to implement this policy.
- A designated health-care professional will be responsible for assessing needs, planning, implementing, evaluating, and periodically updating competency-based training in breastfeeding for all health-care staff dealing with the mother and infant. Such training may differentiate the level of competency required based on staff function and responsibility, including demonstration and documentation of such skills as required.*

Step Three

- Inform all pregnant women about the benefits of breastfeeding.
- Counseling about infant-feeding choices will be made available to pregnant women for whom the hospital provides prenatal care and/or childbirth education. Such counseling will be given in the first trimester, whenever possible.
- The counseling will cover the benefits of breastfeeding (including health benefits to mother and baby), precautions, the advantages of exclusive breastfeeding for the first 4 to 6 months, basic breastfeeding management (including recognition of feeding cues), psychosocial factors and sociocultural barriers influencing decision making (e.g., family support, mother's return to work, diet, etc.), and the mother's individual concerns.

*Asterisk indicates a required criterion for recognition by the U.S. Breastfeeding Health Initiative.

- A current, written description of the content of the counseling will be available for pertinent staff reference.
- The hospital will make information and/or educational materials on breast-feeding available to all health-care professionals/providers for use in pre-natal care and counseling of patients who deliver at the hospital.

Step Four

Offer all mothers the opportunity to initiate breastfeeding within one hour of birth.

- All mothers will be offered their babies to hold with skin-to-skin contact within 30 minutes of birth, unless medically contraindicted.*
- Mothers will be offered help by a staff member to put the baby to the breast, unless medically contraindicated.
- Infant-care procedures will be initiated after the first breastfeed, unless medically contraindicated, and should be conducted at the mother's bedside.

Step Five

Show breastfeeding mothers how to breastfeed and how to maintain lactation, even if they are separated from their infants.

- As soon as possible, and optimally within 3 hours of delivery, health-care professionals will review breastfeeding practices and demonstrate appropriate breastfeeding positioning with the mother and baby.
- Prior to discharge, and as soon as possible after delivery, breastfeeding mothers will be educated on:
  - correct positioning, latch-on, and detachment techniques
  - lactation management for exclusive breastfeeding
  - how to express, handle, and store breastmilk
  - how to sustain lactation if the mother does not choose to exclusively breastfeed.
- Additional individualized assistance to high-risk and special needs mothers and infants, and to mothers who indicate breastfeeding problems, will be provided.

Step Six

Give breastfeeding infants only breastmilk, unless medically contraindicated.

- The hospital will promote breastfeeding as the standard for infant feeding.*
- When a mother requests that her breastfeeding baby be given a breastmilk substitute, the health-care staff will first explore the reasons for the request, address the concerns raised, educate her about the possible consequences to the success of breastfeeding, and document the process and the outcome.
- All educational and promotional materials provided to breastfeeding mothers will be free of overt and/or subtle messages that may decrease the incidence or shorten the duration of breastfeeding.
- Each hospital will review its policy regarding the purchase and distribution of low-cost or free infant formula and assess the impact of the policy on breastfeeding incidence and duration.*

---

*Asterisk indicates a required criterion for recognition by the U.S. Breastfeeding Health Initiative.

Step Seven

Facilitate rooming-in—encourage all mothers and infants to remain together during their hospital stay.

- The health-care staff will encourage and educate mothers about the advantages of having their infants stay with them in the same room.
- The staff will conduct newborn procedures at the mother's bedside and avoid frequent, prolonged absences of newborn from mother.

Step Eight

Encourage unrestricted breastfeeding—when baby exhibits hunger cues or signalsor on request of the mother.

- The nursing staff will be trained to help mothers:
  - understand that babies nurse for a variety of reasons.
  - recognize cues that infants use as a signal of readiness to feed.
  - learn that no restrictions are to be placed on the frequency or length of breastfeeds.
  - understand that babies should be awakened to feed if they sleep too long (8 to 12 feedings every 24 hours is common).

Step Nine

Encourage exclusive sucking at the breast by providing no pacifiers or artificial nipples.

- The designated health-care professional will ensure that, prior to discharge, a responsible staff member explores with each mother, and a support person(s) if she so desires, her plans for infant feeding after discharge.
- When a mother requests that her breastfeeding baby be given an artificial nipple, the health-care staff will first explore the reasons for this request, address the concerns raised and educate her on the possible consequences to the success of breastfeeding, discuss alternative methods of feeding, and document the process and the outcome.
- When a mother requests that her breastfeeding baby be given a pacifier, the health-care staff will first explore the reasons for this request, address the concerns raised and educate her on the possible consequences to the success of breastfeeding, discuss alternative methods of soothing her baby, and document the process and the outcome.

Step Ten

Refer mothers to established breastfeeding and/or mothers' support groups and services, and foster the establishment of those services when they are not available.

- The designated health-care professional will ensure that, prior to discharge, a responsible staff member explores with each mother, and a support person(s) if she so desires, her plans for infant feeding after discharge.

---

*Asterisk indicates a required criterion for recognition by the U.S. Breastfeeding Health Initiative.

• Discharge planning for the mother and infant will include information on available culturally specific support. Examples of support services include: providing a telephone number for call-in and/or names and phone numbers of support organizations or individual resource persons; developing a support group for breastfeeding mothers; scheduling early postdischarge follow-up appointments.*

ESTABLISHMENT AND IMPLEMENTATION OF STATE AND COMMUNITY COALITIONS

Breastfeeding parents should be provided with names and telephone numbers of community-based breastfeeding support groups and lactation professionals they may contact for continuity of lactation education and support. Encouraging the use of various forms of lactation support available in the community is very supportive of a flourishing breastfeeding relationship.

Consult your local directory for possible local breastfeeding support contacts. Social service organizations or listings under the headings of counseling services, health-care services, or children and youth services may provide possible contacts. The following are possible contacts within the community for breastfeeding support and information:

1. Childbirth Education Association
2. Hospital-based breastfeeding professionals
3. Hospital education programs
4. La Leche League
5. Lactation consultants
6. Visiting Nurses' Associations
7. Physicians' offices
8. Public health/WIC agencies
9. Cooperative extension agencies

Many communities have formed breastfeeding coalitions to bring together those individuals interested in promoting, supporting, and protecting breastfeeding. State WIC agencies have been charged by federal guidelines to organize breastfeeding advisory groups in each state to evaluate local efforts and plan supportive activities. Community and state coalitions bring together professionals and consumers from a variety of settings and can be influential in disseminating accurate breastfeeding information. Group-planned activities might include developing community resource lists, creating displays to be used in health fairs and during World Breastfeeding Week, and writing grants to secure financial assistance for community breastfeeding promotion.

---

*Asterisk indicates a required criterion for recognition by the U.S. Breastfeeding Health Initiative.

POST-TEST

For questions 1 to 20, choose the single best answer.

1. A policy that encourages putting the healthy newborn to breast _____ after birth, encourages a successful breastfeeding experience.

   A. 3 hours
   B. the morning
   C. immediately
   D. within two days

2. Showing breastfeeding education videos produced and sponsored by formula companies to women in the hospital or clinic tends to _____ breast-feeding.

   A. encourage
   B. discourage
   C. not affect

3. A policy that encourages _____ feedings for the breast-fed infant encourages a successful breastfeeding experience.

   A. every 4 hours
   B. every 2 to 3 hours during day hours only
   C. on-demand
   D. scheduled according to hospital routine

4. A clinical environment decorated with pictures of women _____ discourages breastfeeding.

   A. breastfeeding
   B. playing with their infants
   C. bottle feeding
   D. none of the above

5. Allowing mothers and infants to remain together throughout the hospital stay is:

   A. rooming-in.
   B. supportive of breastfeeding.
   C. impossible.
   D. both A and B

6. Separating the breastfeeding mother and healthy newborn immediately following birth until after the assessment and bath have taken place _____.

   A. encourages breastfeeding
   B. discourages breastfeeding
   C. has no effect on breastfeeding

7. Ms. Smith notices her client breastfeeding, holding the infant in an "inappropriate" position. She immediately takes the infant from the mother and, while repositioning him, tells the mother "she is doing it all wrong!"

   A. This would encourage breastfeeding.
   B. This would discourage breastfeeding.
   C. This would have no effect on breastfeeding.

8. Offering and/or giving the breastfeeding mother a free formula gift pack on her hospital discharge _____.

    A. encourages breastfeeding
    B. discourages breastfeeding
    C. has no effect on breastfeeding

9. Women seeing _____ infants encourages breastfeeding.

    A. professional health-care workers bottle feeding
    B. mothers breastfeeding their
    C. educational material containing pictures of mothers bottle feeding their
    D. None of the above

10. The health-care staff initiating discussion regarding the woman's intention to breastfeed during the prenatal and postpartum periods encourages breastfeeding.

    A. True
    B. False
    C. Has no effect on breastfeeding

11. The success of a breastfeeding program includes obtaining support and commitment from:

    A. administration.
    B. doctors and nurses.
    C. dietitians and nutrition counselors.
    D. All of the above

12. Policies requiring continued breastfeeding education for all staff coming into contact with women and infants encourage breastfeeding because:

    A. it promotes correct and consistent breastfeeding advise and instructions being given out by staff.
    B. continued education in the area of breastfeeding does not encourage breastfeeding and will have no effect on outcomes.
    C. it ensures that breastfeeding knowledge of staff is up to date with correct and current breastfeeding information.
    D. Both A and C

13. If the breastfeeding relationship must be interrupted, instructions to the mother should include the _____ and _____ of breastmilk.

    A. rest she should obtain; decreasing her supply
    B. expression; storage
    C. nutritional; caloric value
    D. pumping schedule of every 1 to 2 hours while separated from infant; storage

14. Giving breastfed infants water after a nursing session will prevent hyperbilirubinemia.

    A. True
    B. False
    C. All breastfed infants become jaundiced.
    D. Both A and C

15. Policies encouraging and supporting on-demand breastfeedings are ridiculous and unnecessary because:

    A. they will spoil the infant.
    B. they promote overeating and overweight infants.
    C. they are impossible to fit in with the schedule and routine of hospital staff.
    D. None of the above. Policies encouraging and supporting breastfeeding are necessary and encourage a successful and rewarding breastfeeding relationship.

16. Breastfeeding mothers should be given information on community resources they may contact for breastfeeding support and any breastfeeding concerns they may encounter.

    A. True; follow-up and community support can contribute to a successful breastfeeding relationship
    B. False; the breastfeeding mother will receive all of breastfeeding information she needs while in the hospital
    C. True; breastfeeding hurts and is time consuming. The breastfeeding mother will need a shoulder to cry on.

17. Possible community resources for breastfeeding support include:

    A. physician, nurse, and dietitian.
    B. lactation consultant.
    C. WIC program.
    D. La Leche League.
    E. All of the above

18. Information about breastfeeding should be included in all prenatal/childbirth education classes.

    A. True; this allows the pregnant woman to make an informed decision regarding the infant-feeding method she chooses.
    B. False; you don't want to offend anyone.
    C. True; it encourages breastfeeding.
    D. Both A and C

19. Formula, glucose water, or sterile water should not be given to the breastfed infant unless it is medically indicated and ordered by the physician.

    A. True; studies have shown that supplementary or complementary feeds can lead to a diminished milk supply.
    B. False; all breastfed infants need extra nourishment because the mother is never able to produce enough milk to adequately nourish her growing child.
    C. True; frequent breastfeedings can help the mother avoid problems such as engorgement.
    D. Both A and C

20. Which of the following practices and policies are strongly encouraging of successful breastfeeding relationship:

    A. If breastfeeding is not immediately successful, the staff will continue to support and assist the mother.
    B. Breastfeeding mother is given free formula gift kit and infant food literature.
    C. Staff interrupts breastfeeding session for counseling, lab tests, forms to be filled out, etc.
    D. None of the above

SECTION B

Organizational Positions Supportive of Breastfeeding

Jan Simpson, RN, BSN, IBCLC
Rebecca F. Black, MS, RD/LD, IBCLC

LEARNING OBJECTIVES

At the completion of this section, the learner will be able to do the following:

1. Discuss professional positions regarding the promotion of breastfeeding as provided in policy statements.

OUTLINE

I. Professional Position Summaries

    A. American Academy of Pediatrics

    B. American College of Obstetricians and Gynecologists

    C. American Dietetic Association

    D. American Society for Psychoprophylaxis in Obstetrics

    E. Association of Women's Health, Obstetric, and Neonatal Nurses

    F. Breastfeeding Promotion Consortium

    G. Healthy Mothers/Healthy Babies Coalition

    H. Infant Feeding Action Coalition

    I. Institute of Medicine

    J. International Baby Food Action Network

    K. International Board of Lactation Consultant Examiners

    L. International Childbirth Education Association

    M. International Lactation Consultant Association

N. International Organization of Consumer Unions

O. La Leche League International

P. The Maternal and Child Health Interorganizational Nutrition Group

Q. National Association of WIC Directors

R. Special Supplemental Food Program for Women, Infants and Children

S. United Nations Children's Fund

T. World Alliance for Breastfeeding Action

U. World Health Organization

PRE-TEST

For questions 1 to 20, choose the best answer from the following key:

A. True   B. False

1. The American Academy of Pediatrics supports breastfeeding as the "optimal form of infant nutrition."

2. In a statement included in the *Guidelines for Prenatal Care*, the American College of Obstetricians and Gynecologists remarked that "breastfeeding alone can satisfy the infant's nutritional needs for the first four to six months of life."

3. The American Dietetic Association advocates breastfeeding for many reasons, including nutritional, immunologic, physiological, social, and hygienic benefits.

4. The Breastfeeding Promotion Consortium is a breastfeeding mothers' support group that was formed by two breastfeeding mothers in 1956 and now is recognized as an authority on breastfeeding.

5. The IBCLE is a voluntary certification program for individuals desiring to become international board–certified in the field of lactation.

6. La Leche League meetings in communities serve as excellent resources for breastfeeding information for pregnant and lactating women and their families.

7. La Leche League is a national organization reaching breastfeeding families in the United States only.

8. The National Association of WIC Directors believes that breastfeeding should be encouraged as the standard practice of infant feeding by WIC programs throughout the nation.

9. On May 21, 1981, the WHO/UNICEF International Code of Marketing of Breastmilk Substitutes was approved by a vote of 118 to 1. The opposing vote was cast by the United States.

10. The WHO/UNICEF International Code of Marketing of Breastmilk Substitutes was developed with the goal of banning all sales of infant formulas and all education about the products for members of the medical community.

11. The WIC program is a governmental agency that functions only as a formula distributor in the United States.

12. The WIC program is a governmental agency that strives to improve the nutrition of pregnant and lactating women, infants, and children less than five years of age who meet eligibility criteria.

13. AWHONN, formerly NAACOG, recognizes the importance of the nurse's role in promoting and supporting the lactation process through her own continued education in the field of lactation.

14. The International Lactation Consultant Association is an association that provides current breastfeeding information and support for lactation consultants and other professionals in the health-care field interested in breastfeeding.

15. The promotion and protection of breastfeeding to WIC clientele is an important priority within the WIC program.

16. The Healthy Mothers/Healthy Babies Coalition's purpose is provide infants and their mothers with health check-ups on a regular basis.

17. The Healthy Mothers/Healthy Babies Coalition's purpose is the promotion of prenatal and infant care, including the promotion of breastfeeding.

18. The International Lactation Consultant Association publishes the *Journal of Human Lactation*, a periodical of scientific and clinical findings, case studies, and discussions of information pertinent to the practice of lactation consultants.

19. The position of the National Association of WIC Directors is that all WIC personnel should promote and support the continued breastfeeding relationship in order to increase breastfeeding incidence and duration among WIC clients.

20. The WHO/UNICEF International Code of Marketing of Breastmilk Substitutes was developed with the intent that it would be adopted by governments to protect the health of infants by preventing inappropriate marketing of breastmilk substitutes.

Professional Position Summaries

The following sections contain brief summaries and excerpts from position papers on infant nutrition provided by various professional health-care organizations.

AMERICAN ACADEMY OF PEDIATRICS

"The primary goal of the American Academy of Pediatrics (AAP) is to encourage optimal infant nutrition through the promotion of breastfeeding, stressing the superiority of human milk and the proper use of nutritionally appropriate breast-milk substitutes for infants who cannot be breast-fed" (AAP, 1982).

Since its beginning, the American Academy of Pediatrics has supported breast-feeding as the "optimal form of infant nutrition." Recommendations by the Academy have promoted breastfeeding as the "foundation of good feeding practices" through the years. According to AAP (1976):

Important steps which will encourage breastfeeding include more educational programs for adolescents and pregnant women and reinforcement by obstetricians, pediatricians and nurses attending pregnant women. Changes in employment policies and working conditions and provision of daycare centers at or near places of employment to make breastfeeding practical for working mothers will increase the frequency of breastfeeding. Such changes are urgently needed where rural poor have migrated to urban areas in the United States and elsewhere.

Another excerpt from the Academy's policy statement on the promotion of breast-feeding discusses a 1978 joint publication of the AAP and the Canadian Paediatric Society entitled *Breastfeeding: A Commentary in Celebration of the International Year of the Child*. This publication provided up-to-date information concerning the benefits of breastfeeding to infants. In 1980, AAP issued a follow-up statement proposing ways to execute the recommendations it had given to encourage the breastfeeding relationship:

Physicians, nurses, nursing personnel and hospitals need to examine their practices and procedures that encourage or discourage breastfeeding. The cultural attitudes and life styles of today's world tend to mitigate against breastfeeding. Yet the benefits of breastfeeding to the neonate and the mother are so numerous that pediatricians must strongly encourage the practice.

In the June 1992 issue of *Pediatrics*, the AAP Committee on Nutrition published the statement "The Use of Whole Cow's Milk in Infancy." It reinforces the position that infants be fed breastmilk for the first 6 to 12 months.

In the April 1993 *AAP News,* the association published its policy on formula advertising directly to the public. The following is excerpted:

The AAP reaffirms its support for breastfeeding as the best and most appropriate form of infant feeding; further, the AAP reaffirms its opposition to the direct advertising of formula to the public because of the negative effect such advertising might have on the practice of breastfeeding. The AAP reserves the right to continue to speak out against direct advertising of infant formula and other practices that might be deleterious to successful breastfeeding.

The third edition of *Guidelines for Perinatal Care* was released in April 1992. This publication is jointly sponsored by the American College of Obstetricians and

Gynecologists and the American Academy of Pediatrics. The guidelines discuss medical support for lactation under normal circumstances.

AMERICAN COLLEGE OF OBSTETRICIANS AND GYNECOLOGISTS

The American College of Obstetricians and Gynecologists (ACOG) presented a statement (in the 1988 second edition of *Guidelines for Perinatal Care*) recommending that "mothers be encouraged to breastfeed" and that "breastfeeding alone can satisfy the infant's nutritional needs for the first four to six months of life."

The ACOG has also promoted the discussion of breastfeeding by the obstetrician/gynecologist (OB/GYN) with patients, preferably both prospective parents, before becoming pregnant or early in the pregnancy. Their guidelines were reaffirmed by the American Academy of Pediatrics and the American College of Obstetricians and Gynecologists in 1992 in the third edition of the *Guidelines for Perinatal Care*.

AMERICAN DIETETIC ASSOCIATION

The position paper adopted by the American Dietetic Association (ADA) in 1986, "Promotion of Breastfeeding," discusses the benefits of breastfeeding to both the mother and infant, as well as documents the nutritional advantages of breastmilk. It strongly encourages members of the ADA to participate in encouraging and supporting breastfeeding. This policy was reaffirmed in 1991 by the House of Delegates of ADA and published in the April 1993 *Journal of the American Dietetic Association*:

The American Dietetic Association advocates breastfeeding because of the nutritional and immunologic benefits of human milk for the infant, the physiological, social, and hygienic benefits of the breastfeeding process for the mother and infant, and the economic benefits to the family and health-care system.

AMERICAN SOCIETY FOR PSYCHOPROPHYLAXIS IN OBSTETRICS

The American Society for Psychoprophylaxis in Obstetrics (ASPO/Lamaze) sponsors prenatal classes in the Lamaze/psychoprohylaxis method of prepared childbirth for expectant couples. In April 1992, ASPO/Lamaze adopted the WHO International Code of Marketing of Breastmilk Substitutes and issued a position paper supporting breastfeeding. The organization distributed the ILCA publication, *Summary of the Hazards of Infant Formula* to its members in 1993.

ASSOCIATION OF WOMEN'S HEALTH, OBSTETRIC, AND NEONATAL NURSES

The Association of Women's Health, Obstetric, and Neonatal Nurses (AWHONN), formerly NAACOG, the Organization for Obstetric, Gynecologic and Neonatal

Nurses, approved its position statement on the issue of breastfeeding in 1992 (AWHONN, 1992). It states that "AWHONN recognizes the many benefits of breast-feeding and advocates breastfeeding as the optimal method of infant feeding."

The AWHONN statement discusses the importance of educating the public so that informed choices regarding infant feeding can be made, as well as the importance of the nurse's role in promoting and supporting the lactation process through her own continued education in the field of lactation. "AWHONN supports the belief that the promotion of breastfeeding will contribute to the reduction of infant morbidity and mortality rates" (AWHONN, 1992).

BREASTFEEDING PROMOTION CONSORTIUM

The purpose of the Breastfeeding Promotion Consortium (BPC) is to promote breastfeeding collaboratively. Meeting semi-annually, the BPC is an organization that was formed by the U.S. Department of Agriculture (USDA) in 1991. It consists of members from the following national organizations:

1. American Academy of Family Physicians
2. American Academy of Pediatrics
3. American College of Obstetricians and Gynecologists
4. American Hospital Association
5. American Nurses Association
6. Association of Maternal and Child Health Programs
7. Center on Budget and Policy Priorities
8. Healthy Mothers, Healthy Babies Coalition
9. House Select Committee on Hunger
10. La Leche League International
11. National Association of Pediatric Nurse Associates and Practitioners
12. National Association of WIC Directors
13. Association of Women's Health, Obstetric, and Neonatal Nurses
14. U.S. Department of Health and Human Services, Maternal and Child Health Bureau
15. U.S. Department of Agriculture

The BPC has agreed to join the USDA in working toward the following goals: (1) to increase knowledge and awareness among the general population of breastfeeding as the optimal method of infant feeding, and (2) to help create a positive public climate with respect to the acceptability of breastfeeding.

HEALTHY MOTHERS/HEALTHY BABIES COALITION

The Healthy Mothers/Healthy Babies (HMHB) Coalition combines representatives of the U.S. Department of Agriculture and Department of Health and Human Services (USDHHS) and other public and private organizations. Its purpose is the promotion of prenatal and infant care, including the promotion of breastfeeding. HMHB coalitions in many areas have received public and private finding for breastfeeding promotion projects.

In 1989, the Florida Healthy Mothers/Healthy Babies Coalition developed a statewide committee composed of La Leche League representatives, WIC representatives, a coalition of Florida childbirth educators, the Florida AWHONN, and various members of the lay community. The goal of this committee was to develop model breastfeeding policies for use by Florida hospitals (Breunig & Brady, 1992). After much research and review, 13 model hospital policies were developed with the goals of:

- Increasing the incidence of breastfeeding through a positive and supportive environment.
- Promoting the distribution of consistent breastfeeding information to mothers.
- Providing accurate and up-to-date breastfeeding information.

In addition, the committee published a training program for hospital staff—*Model Hospital Policies and Protocols to Support Breastfeeding Mothers* (Breunig & Merwin, 1990).

The national HMHB Coalition recently completed an 18-month feasibility study of WHO/UNICEFs Baby Friendly Hospital Initiative (HMHB, 1994). The study was sponsored through the Maternal and Child Health Bureau of the U.S. Department of Health and Human Services. See U.S. Breastfeeding Health Initiative in section A of this chapter for the results of this study.

INFANT FEEDING ACTION COALITION

The Infant Feeding Action Coalition (INFACT) is a nonprofit, nongovernmental, voluntary organization in Canada that was developed in response to the International Code of Marketing of Breastmilk Substitutes adopted by the WHO. INFACT promotes better maternal and infant health by protecting breastfeeding and supporting appropriate maternal and infant nutrition.

INFACT is active in researching, developing, and producing educational resources for health-care professionals and lay persons. They also observe and evaluate the marketing practices of the Canadian infant-food industry. INFACT's endeavors include influencing Canada's governmental policy in relation to the protection and promotion of breastfeeding as they lobby for full execution of the WHO/UNICEF international code.

INSTITUTE OF MEDICINE

The Institute of Medicine (IOM) of the National Academy of Sciences (NAS) includes the committee Nutritional Status During Pregnancy and Lactation and subcommittee Nutrition During Lactation. These two committees are comprised of experts from fields such as nutritional sciences, obstetrics and gynecology, pediatrics, and community medicine. Several Institute of Medicine publications pertinent to lactation specialists are: *Nutrition Services in Perinatal Care* (1992), *Nutrition During Pregnancy* (1990), *Nutrition During Lactation* (1991), and *Nutrition During Pregnancy and Lactation: An Implementation Guide* (1992).

INTERNATIONAL BABY FOOD ACTION NETWORK

The International Baby Food Action Network (IBFAN) was founded by the International Organization of Consumer Unions (IOCU) and is a coalition of voluntary organizations that endeavor to improve child health and nutrition by fostering breastfeeding and eliminating the marketing of breastmilk substitutes. IBFAN is working in developing countries as well as industrialized nations and consists of 140 groups in 74 countries (IBFAN/IOCU, 1990).

IBFAN was instrumental in the development of the WHO/UNICEF International Code of Marketing of Breastmilk Substitutes. They are continuing to see that marketing practices throughout the world change appropriately in response to the code.

INTERNATIONAL BOARD OF LACTATION CONSULTANT EXAMINERS

The International Board of Lactation Consultant Examiners (IBLCE©) is a voluntary, international certification program for lactation consultants. It is a nonprofit corporation that was developed to administer a certification program for individuals desiring to become board-certified internationally in the field of lactation. The certification by examination was established based on guidelines that were developed by the National Commission for Certifying Agencies.

Certification allows the lactation consultant to use the title of IBCLC© (International Board Certified Lactation Consultant) and validates the special skills and knowledge for employers, colleagues, and consumers. A goal of this certification process is to improve health care and establish standards for lactation consultants.

To be accepted to sit for the certification exam, the applicant must apply and meet eligibility requirements. Additional information and location of exam sites may be obtained by writing to the IBLCE© (IBLCE, 1996). See Section C in this chapter for the address and phone number.

INTERNATIONAL CHILDBIRTH EDUCATION ASSOCIATION

The International Childbirth Education Association (ICEA) position paper on infant feeding was written and published by the International Lactation Consultants Association in February 1991 and adopted by the ICEA in December 1991. It states: "The International Childbirth Education Association affirms the right of all women to breastfeed their babies, of all babies to receive human milk, and of all men and women to assist mothers in protecting these rights."

ICEA encourages them to breastfeed by furnishing information and resources to breastfeeding women. ICEA acknowledges that breastfeeding is a choice, hence they provide knowledge on breastfeeding as well as bottle feeding (ICEA, 1992).

INTERNATIONAL LACTATION CONSULTANT ASSOCIATION

The International Lactation Consultant Association (ILCA) is the professional association for lactation consultants. Founded in 1985, ILCA provides current breastfeeding information and support for lactation consultants and other professionals in the health-care field who are interested in breastfeeding. ILCA serves as an advisory body for authorities with responsibility for health of mothers and infants. ILCA hosts an annual international breastfeeding conference for lactation consultants each year and publishes the *Journal of Human Lactation* quarterly.

ILCA's position paper on infant feeding confronts common practices that occur which are not supportive of breastfeeding and invites research into other areas. It was written and published in February 1991 and states: "The International Lactation Consultant Association affirms the right of all women to breastfeed their babies, of all babies to receive human milk, and of all men and women to assist mothers in protecting these rights."

ILCA's position paper also includes 44 key points of recent breastfeeding research and clinical applications of the findings. Recognizing the importance of breastfeeding research and remaining current with breastfeeding information, ILCA requires that their position paper be reviewed and updated on a regular basis (ILCA, 1991).

INTERNATIONAL ORGANIZATION OF CONSUMER UNIONS

An independent nonprofit foundation, begun in 1972, the International Organization of Consumer Unions (IOCU) is a federation of consumer organizations dedicated to the protection and promotion of consumer rights worldwide through information, research, and education activities. The IOCU connects the activities of 170 consumer organizations in 70 countries and was instrumental in the publication of *Protecting Infant Health: A Health Worker's Guide to the International Code of Marketing of Breastmilk Substitutes* (IBFAN/IOCU, 1990).

LA LECHE LEAGUE INTERNATIONAL

La Leche League International (LLLI) is a worldwide organization internationally recognized as an authority on breastfeeding. It reaches over 46 countries. Two breastfeeding mothers, Mary White and Marian Thompson, founded this breastfeeding mothers' support group in 1956.

Local chapters of LLLI hold informal meetings in communities, with breastfeeding mothers and their children attending, as well as pregnant women. An accredited La Leche League leader presents educational topics focused on various aspects of the breastfeeding relationship at each meeting. Practical breastfeeding tips and many other parenting tips are also exchanged by the leader and group participants. The leaders are available for breastfeeding assistance between scheduled meetings on a voluntary basis. Over 9,000 volunteer LLLI leaders assist more than 100,000 families in the United States each year (Riordan & Auerbach, 1993).

La Leche League's mission statement reiterates that their purpose is:

- To help the mother learn to breastfeed her baby;
- To encourage good mothering through breastfeeding, thereby stimulating the optimal physical and emotional growth of the child and the development of a close family relationship;
- To promote a better understanding of the values of breastfeeding, parenting, childbirth, and related subjects;
- To offer discussion meetings and conduct lectures on the purposes stated above and on related subjects for such educational purposes as are herein expressed.

La Leche League International's publication for lay people, *The Womanly Art of Breastfeeding,* is available in six languages (LLLI, 1991). LLLI also publishes *The Breastfeeding Answer Book* for professionals (Mohrbacher & Stock, 1996). Many of the league's informative breastfeeding pamphlets are available in 34 languages. A list of translated materials is available free of charge by contacting LLLI.

La Leche League International sponsors a physician workshop and an international meeting for lactation educators, league leaders, and parents. Regional meetings for league leaders are also offered. Also, a one-day program travels to six locations annually. Recent efforts include the development of peer-counselor training as support groups for various ethnic and economic groups and continue to gain in popularity and effectiveness.

MATERNAL AND CHILD HEALTH INTERORGANIZATIONAL NUTRITION GROUP

The Maternal and Child Health Interorganizational Nutrition Group (MCHING) consists of various national organizations; the following are currently members:

- American Dietetic Association
- American Public Health Association
- Association of Faculties of Graduate Programs in Public Health Nutrition
- Association of Maternal and Child Health Programs
- Society for Nutrition Education

On December 6 through 8, 1990, the MCHING held a national workshop, Call to Action: Better Nutrition for Mothers, Children, and Families, convened in Washington, DC. The workshop provided a chance for many agencies and organizations to join together in developing an action plan to improve maternal and child nutrition services. Recommendations, actions, and strategies were developed. Excerpts from the 1990 MCHING recommendations developed are listed here:

Recommendation 5—"Educate and train all health-care providers, both professional and paraprofessional, working with or planning to work with pregnant women, infants, children, adolescents, and families on sound infant and child feeding practices, including breastfeeding."

Recommendation 8 and Recommendation 11—"Promote breastfeeding among all women to achieve the year 2000 National Health Promotion and Disease Prevention Objectives for breastfeeding, and establish breastfeeding as the societal norm for infant feeding."

Recommendation 12—"Develop a U.S. Infant Feeding Code which positively states the responsibilities of formula and food manufacturing industries regarding their role in promoting breastfeeding and appropriate infant feeding practices."

Recommendation 13—"Generate reliable and standardized data on infant feeding practices, including breastfeeding. Such data should provide information about service delivery as well as outcomes related to infant feeding."

In response to the MCHING recommendations, the Maternal and Child Health Bureau of the USDA is currently funding breastfeeding projects in 16 states. These projects are all working toward achieving the year 2000 objectives for the nation: 75% of mothers initiate breastfeeding and 50% of mothers continue breastfeeding at 5 to 6 months postpartum.

NATIONAL ASSOCIATION OF WIC DIRECTORS

The position of the National Association of WIC Directors (NAWD) on the promotion of breastfeeding in WIC programs is as follows:

As health professionals have a responsibility to provide services designed to optimize the health of their clients, WIC health professionals are committed to encouraging breastfeeding as the preferred method of infant feeding. Therefore, the National Association of WIC Directors calls for all WIC state and local agencies to aggressively promote breastfeeding (NAWD, 1989).

In addition, NAWD's position paper on breastfeeding discusses how breastfeeding should be instituted as the standard practice of infant feeding in WIC programs throughout the nation. The paper also states that all WIC personnel should promote and support the continued breastfeeding relationship in order to increase breastfeeding incidence and duration among the WIC population.

SPECIAL SUPPLEMENTAL NUTRITION PROGRAM FOR WOMEN, INFANTS AND CHILDREN

The Special Supplemental Nutrition Program for Women, Infants and Children (WIC) is a governmental agency striving to improve the nutrition of pregnant and lactating women, infants, and children under the age of five in the United States. The program provides free nutrition counseling and food supplements, including breastmilk substitutes, to low-income mothers and their infants who meet eligibility requirements.

Since the 1980s, the promotion and protection of breastfeeding for clientele has become an important priority within the WIC program. The women enrolled in the WIC program tend to be the part of the population that has proven to be the least likely to breastfeed. Mothers who choose to breastfeed are provided with more food for themselves and their benefits of enrollment continue for one year (instead of the six months for nonbreastfeeders). Various WIC programs provide lactation counseling from trained health-care staff, and many have hired lactation consultants specifically for this promotional task. WIC funds allow for the continued education of its health-care workers with respect to breastfeeding, as well as promotional and informative breastfeeding materials to be given out to clientele. Since 1991, WIC has enforced a strict ban on all items displayed or used within the WIC clinic setting that has any name or form of breastmilk substitute advertisement on it. Guidelines also require that breastmilk substitutes be stored in closets or cabinets, out of view of clients.

UNITED NATIONS CHILDREN'S FUND

The United Nations Children's Fund (UNICEF) promotes and supports breastfeeding. UNICEF continues its support of the national efforts to reduce the occurrence of inappropriate bottle-feeding practices while advocating compliance with the International Code of Marketing of Breastmilk Substitutes (Jelliffe & Jelliffe, 1988).

In 1985, UNICEF received worldwide coverage on its *State of the World's Children* report, which recognized the superiority of breastfeeding and was endorsed by leaders around the world. The report states:

As more and more studies show that the change from breast to bottle can double and triple the risk to the child's life and growth, so it becomes clear that the campaign to promote and protect breastfeeding is as vital as any of the other low-cost strategies now available to protect the health and normal growth of children in poor communities (UNICEF, 1985, p. 3).

U.S. COMMITTEE FOR UNICEF

While study of the BFHI for the United States was being conducted, the U.S. Committee for UNICEF began offering Certificates of Intent and technical assistance to hospitals willing to commit to the global Ten Steps of the BFHI. In addition to awarding the certificates in collaboration with the Vanderbilt University School of Nursing, the committee conducted in-depth telephone interviews with 75 of the first hospitals in the United States to receive the Certificates of Intent. As a result of these interviews, the committee published *Barriers and Solutions to the Global Ten Steps to Successful Breastfeeding: A Summary of In-Depth Interviews with Hospitals Participating in the WHO/UNICEF Baby Friendly Hospital Initiative Interim Program in the United States*. This report outlines each of the ten steps, identifies barriers, and presents solutions to overcoming them. The document can be ordered from the U.S. Committee for UNICEF, Office of Public Policy and Government Relations, 110 Maryland Avenue, N.E., Box 36, Washington, DC 20002.

WORLD ALLIANCE FOR BREASTFEEDING ACTION

The World Alliance for Breastfeeding Action (WABA) is a group of national and international organizations dedicated to the promotion of breastfeeding. WABA was developed in response to the Innocenti Declaration of February 15, 1991. It was formed to act on the worldwide initiative set forth by the joint WHO/UNICEF statement *Protecting, Promoting and Supporting Breastfeeding: The Special Role of Maternity Services*. The important tasks taken on by WABA include the coordination and exchange of information between organizations and countries, mobilizing support for breastfeeding programs, and monitoring implementation of breast-feeding codes. WABA recognizes that "breastfeeding is a basic human right of all children and mothers" (WABA, 1992).

WORLD HEALTH ORGANIZATION

The World Health Organization (WHO) regards breastfeeding as the ideal way of providing the perfect and superior nutrition for infants. They recognize the multiple benefits breastfeeding offers the infant as well as the nursing mother (WHO, 1990).

A significant portion of the maternal and child health nutrition programs of the World Health Organization are focused on the promotion of breastfeeding and sound weaning practices. WHO supports research on identifying and examining the determinants of infant- and young child-feeding practices and care. WHO believes that increasing the incidence and duration of breastfeeding by furthering the education of health-care and social service workers and mothers is a significant and necessary part of national health and social programs (Jelliffe & Jelliffe, 1988).

WHO continues its work in cooperation with UNICEF in the promotion of breast-feeding, as it has for many years. WHO and UNICEF believe that "health-care practices, particularly those related to the care of mothers and newborn infants, stand out as one of the most promising means of increasing the prevalence and duration of breastfeeding" (WHO/UNICEF, 1989).

The International Code of Marketing of Breastmilk Substitutes was passed at the Fifteenth Plenary Meeting of the WHO in 1981. The only dissenting vote was cast by the United States (WHO, 1981). The WHO reaffirmed the code in 1994; the United States voted for the code at this meeting (WHO, 1994).

POST-TEST

For questions 1 to 20, choose the best answer from the following key:

A. True   B. False

1. The promotion and protection of breastfeeding to WIC clientele is an important priority within the WIC program.

2. The Healthy Mothers/Healthy Babies Coalition's purpose is the promotion of prenatal and infant care, including the promotion of breastfeeding.

3. The IBCLE is a voluntary certification program for individuals desiring to become international board-certified in the field of lactation.

4. The American Dietetic Association advocates breastfeeding for many reasons, including the nutritional, immunologic, physiological, social, hygienic, and economic benefits.

5. The WIC program is a governmental agency that functions only as a formula distributor in the United States.

6. The National Association of WIC Directors believes that breastfeeding should be encouraged as the standard practice of infant feeding by WIC programs throughout the nation.

7. The WHO International Code of Marketing of Breastmilk Substitutes was developed with the intent that it would be adopted by governments to protect the health of infants by preventing inappropriate marketing of breastmilk substitutes.

8. The International Lactation Consultant Association is an association that provides current breastfeeding information and support for lactation consultants and other professionals in the health-care field interested in breastfeeding.

9. AWHONN, formerly NAACOG, recognizes the importance of the nurse's role in promoting and supporting the lactation process through continued education in the field of lactation.

10. The Breastfeeding Promotion Consortium is a breastfeeding mothers' support group that was formed by two breastfeeding mothers in 1956 and now is recognized as an authority on breastfeeding.

11. In a statement included in the *Guidelines for Perinatal Care*, the American College of Obstetricians and Gynecologists remarked that "breastfeeding alone can satisfy the infant's nutritional needs for the first four to six months of life."

12. On May 21, 1981, the WHO/UNICEF International Code of Marketing of Breastmilk Substitutes was approved by a vote of 118 to 1. The opposing vote was cast by the United States.

13. The American Academy of Pediatrics supports breastfeeding as the "optimal form of infant nutrition."

14. La Leche League meetings in communities serve as excellent resources for breastfeeding information for pregnant and lactating women and their families.

15. The WHO International Code of Marketing of Breastmilk Substitutes was developed with the goal of banning all sales of infant formulas and all education about the products for members of the medical community.

16. The position of the National Association of WIC Directors states that all WIC personnel should promote and support the continued breastfeeding relationship to increase the breastfeeding incidence and duration among WIC clients.

17. La Leche League is a national organization reaching breastfeeding families in the United States only.

18. The Healthy Mothers/Healthy Babies Coalition's purpose is to provide infants and their mothers with health check-ups on a regular basis.

19. The WIC program is a governmental agency that strives to improve the nutrition of pregnant and lactating women, infants, and children less than five years of age who meet eligibility criteria.

20. The International Lactation Consultant Association publishes the *Journal of Human Lactation*, a periodical of scientific and clinical findings, case studies, and discussions of information pertinent to the practice of lactation consultants.

SECTION C

Breastfeeding Resources

Jan Simpson, RN, BSN, IBCLC
Rebecca F. Black, MS, RD/LD, IBCLC

LEARNING OBJECTIVES

At the completion of this section, the learner will be able to do the following:

1. Contact various breastfeeding resources for educational information, materials, and publications.

Academy of Breastfeeding Medicine (ABM)
(organization for physicians)
601 Elmwood Ave., Box 777
Rochester, NY 14642
Phone: 716-275-4354
Fax: 716-461-3614
RLAW@neonat.pediatrics.rochester.edu

ALMA Seminars and Publications
P.O. Box 39
Wendouree, Victoria 3355
Australia

ALMA/NMAA Lactation Resource Centre
5 St. George's Rd., Armadale
Melbourne, Victoria 3143
Australia
Phone: 61-3-9576-0829
Fax: 61-3-9576-0829

Ameda Egnell
755 Industrial Dr.
Cary, IL 60013
Phone: 800-323-8750 / 847-639-2900
Fax: 847-639-7895

American Academy of Pediatrics
141 Northwest Point Blvd.
P.O. Box 927
Elk Grove Village, IL 60009-0927
Phone: 708-228-5005
Fax: 847-228-5097
Kidsdoc@AAP.org

**American College of Obstetricians
and Gynecologists**
409 12th St., S.W.
Washington, DC 20024-2188
Phone: 202-638-5577
Fax: 202-484-5107

American Dietetic Association
216 West Jackson Blvd., Suite 800
Chicago, IL 60606-6995
Phone: 312-899-0040
Fax: 312-899-4845
http://www.eatright.org

American Medical Association
515 North State St.
Chicago, IL 60610
Phone: 312-464-5471
Fax: 312-464-5842

American Public Health Association
1015 15th St., N.W., Suite 300
Washington, DC 20005
Phone: 202-789-5600
Fax: 202-789-5661

Association for Breastfeeding Fashions
P.O. Box 4378
Sunland, CA 91040
Phone: 818-352-0697

**Association of Women's Health, Obstetric
and Neonatal Nurses (AWHONN)**
700 14th St., N.W., Suite 600
Washington, DC 20005
Phone: 202-662-1600
Fax: 202-737-0575

ASPO/Lamaze
1200 19th St., N.W., Suite 300
Washington, DC 20036-2422
Phone: 800-368-4404 / 202-857-1128
Fax: 202-223-4579
ASPO@FBA.com

Augusta Nutrition Consultants, Inc.
4571-A Cox Rd.
Evans, GA 30809
Phone: 706-860-8935
Fax: 706-860-8932
reblack@augusta.net

The B.E.S.T. Connection
23 Messalonskee Ave.
Waterville, ME 04901
Phone: 207-877-9109

Best Start
3500 East Fletcher Ave., Suite 519
Tampa, FL 33613
Phone: 800-277-4975 / 813-971-2119
Fax: 813-971-2280

blis™ Prolac, Inc.
P.O. Box 130
Skaneateles, NY 13152
Phone: 800-625-2547 / 315-685-1955
Fax: 315-685-0447

**Boston Association for Childbirth Education/
Nursing Mother's Council**
P.O. Box 29
Newtonville, MA 02160
Phone: 617-244-5102

Bravado Designs
68 Broadview Ave.
Toronto, Ontario M4M 2E6
Canada
Phone: 416-466-8652

Breastfeeding—A Parent's Guide
P.O. Box 501046
Atlanta, GA 31150-1046
Phone: 770-913-9332
Fax: 770-913-0822

The Breastfeeding Center at Crozer-Chester Medical Center
One Medical Center Blvd.
Upland, PA 19013
Phone: 610-447-2744

Breastfeeding Connection
618 North Wheaton Ave.
Wheaton, IL 60187
Phone: 708-665-6848
Fax: 708-260-8879
IBCLC@AOL.com

Breastfeeding Mothers' Support Group
7 Jalan Novena Selatan
Singapore 308562
Phone: 2513116
Fax: 2513116

Breastfeeding Promotion Consortium
U.S. Department of Agriculture
FNS/OAE–Room 214 POC
Washington, DC 20250
Phone: 202-727-3155

Breastfeeding Resource Center
Mercy Health Center
4300 W. Memorial Rd.
Oklahoma City, OK 73120
Phone: 405-752-3282

Breastfeeding Resources
4340 Young Rd.
Syracuse, NY 13215
Phone: 315-492-6437

Breastfeeding Support Consultants
228 Park Lane
Chalfont, PA 18914
Phone: 215-822-1281
Fax: 215-997-7879
bsccenter@AOL.com

Breastfeeding Support Network
330 S. Eagle St.
Oshkosh, WI 54904
Phone: 414-231-1611
Fax: 414-231-1697

Center for Breastfeeding Information/ La Leche League Int.
P.O. Box 1209
Franklin Park, IL 60131-8209
Phone: 847-455-7730

Center to Prevent Childhood Malnutrition
7200 Wisconsin Ave., Suite 204
Bethesda, MD 20814
Phone: 301-986-5777
Fax: 817-751-0221

Childbirth Graphics
P.O. Box 21207
Waco, TX 76702-1207
Phone: 800-299-3366, ext. 287
http://www.WRSGroup.com

Child Survival Action News
1101 Connecticut Ave., N.W., Suite 605
Washington, DC 20006

Clearinghouse on Infant Feeding and Maternal Nutrition/American Public Health Association
1015 15th St., N.W., Suite 300
Washington, DC 20005
Phone: 202-789-5600
Fax: 202-789-5661

Compleat Mother and Friends of Breastfeeding Society
P.O. Box 209
Minot, ND 58702
Phone: 701-852-2822
Fax: 701-852-2822

Department of Health Promotion Clinical Services Institute/University College
Galway, Ireland
Phone: 353-91-524411, ext. 3466
Fax: 353-91-750547

Douglas College Continuing Education
P.O. Box 2503
New Westminister, BC V3L 5B2
Canada
Phone: 604-527-5045
Fax: 604-527-5155

Eastern Pennsylvania Milk Bank
P.O. Box 3262
Bethlehem, PA 18017
Phone: 610-691-6462

Evergreen Hospital Medical Center
12040 N.E. 128 St.
Mailstop #37
Kirkland, WA 98034
Phone: 206-899-3486
Fax: 206-899-3488

Family Health International
P.O. Box 13950
Research Triangle Park, NC 27709
Phone: 919-544-7040
Fax: 206-899-3488
http://www.skhalas@fhi.org

Florida Healthy Mothers/Healthy Babies Coalition
15 S.E. First Ave.
Suite A
Gainesville, FL 32601

For Zealots Only
Bright Future Lactation Resource Center
6540 Cedarview Ct.
Dayton, OH 45459-1214
Phone: 800-667-8939/513-438-9458
Fax: 513-438-3229

Four Dee Products
6014 Lattimer
Houston, TX 77035
Phone: 713-261-2291

Geddes Productions
10546 McVine Ave.
Sunland, CA 91040
Phone: 818-951-2809

Georgetown University Medical Center
3800 Reservoir Rd., N.W.
Washington, DC 20007
Phone: 202-784-6455
Fax: 202-784-2505

Global Graffiti
P.O. Box 708
Evans, GA 30809
Phone: 706-869-1653

Grant MacEwan Community College
Health and Community Studies
P.O. Box 1796
Edmonton, Alberta T5J 2P2
Canada
Phone: 403-497-5717
Fax: 403-497-5170

Health Education Associates, Inc.
8 Jan Sebastian Way
Sandwich, MA 02563
Phone: 508-888-8044
Fax: 508-888-8050

Healthy People 2000: National Health Promotion and Disease Prevention Objectives
Superintendent of Documents
Government Printing Office
Washington, DC 20402
Phone: 202-783-3238

Human Lactation Center
666 Sturges Highway
Westport, CT 06880

Human Milk Banking Association of North America
P.O. Box 370464
West Hartford, CT 06137-0464
Phone: 203-232-8809
Fax: 860-232-0113
lahmbana@tiac.net

Infant Feeding Action Coalition (INFACT)
Contact: INFACT Canada
10 Trinity Square
Toronto, Ontario M5G 1B1
Canada
Phone: 416-595-9819

Institute for Reproductive Health
Georgetown University Medical Center
2115 Wisconsin Ave., N.W.
Suite 602
Washington, DC 20007
Phone: 202-687-1392
Fax: 202-687-6846

International Baby Food Action Network (IBFAN)
Contact: IBFAN North America
212 Third Ave. N.
Suite 300
Minneapolis, MN 55401

International Board of Lactation Consultant Examiners (IBLCE©)
P.O. Box 2348
Falls Church, VA 22042
Phone: 703-560-7332

International Childbirth Education Association (ICEA)
P.O. Box 20048
Minneapolis, MN 55420
Phone: 612-854-8660

International Lactation Consultant Association (ILCA)
200 North Michigan Ave.
Suite 300
Chicago, IL 60601-3821
Phone: 312-541-1710
Fax: 312-541-1271
71005.1134@Compuserve.com

International Organization of Consumer Unions (IOCU)
Regional Office for Asia
and the Pacific
P.O. Box 1045
Penang, Malaysia

Jones and Bartlett Publishers
40 Tall Pine Dr.
Sudbury, MA 01776
Phone: 800-832-0034/508-443-5000
Fax: 508-443-8000

Lact-Aid
P.O. Box 1066
Athens, TN 37371
Phone: 423-744-9090
laljl@MSN.com

Lactation Associates
254 Conant Rd.
Weston, MA 02193
Phone: 617-893-3553
Fax: 617-893-8608
marshalact@AOL.com

The Lactation Center and Mothers' Milk Bank
Presbyterian/St. Luke's Medical Center
1740 South Limestone
Lexington, KY 40503
Phone: 606-275-6502

The Lactation Clinic, Inc. and Childbearing Family Center
401 South Green Rd.
Cleveland, OH 44121

Lactation Consultant Services
11320 Shady Glen Rd.
Oklahoma City, OK 73162
Phone: 405-722-2163

Lactation Consultant Services
111 Pilgrims Way
Kemsing
Kent TN15 6TE
England
Phone: 0585-493873

Lactation Institute and Breastfeeding Clinic
16430 Ventura Blvd.
Suite 303
Encino, CA 91436-2125
Phone: 818-995-1913
Fax: 818-981-9042

Lactation Seminars, Inc.
10316 Sunstrem Lane
Boca Raton, FL 33428
Phone: 407-482-2670
Fax: 407-482-2670

Lactation Supportive Service
British Columbia Children's Hospital
Vancouver, BC V6H 3V4
Canada
Phone: 604-875-2345, ext. 7607

Lactation Training Team
8 Pinegrove Rd.
Swords
Dublin, Ireland
Phone: 01-8403349

LACT-ED, Inc.
5095 Olentangy River Rd.
Columbus, OH 43235-3440
Phone: 614-459-6313
Fax: 614-538-9566

Lactnet
For connection to this on-line
service for lactation supporters,
contact Kathleen Bruce at her
e-mail address: kbruce@together.net

La Leche League International, Inc.
1400 N. Meacham Rd.
P.O. Box 4079
Schaumburg, IL 60168-4079
Phone: 847-519-7730
Fax: 847-519-0035

Lansinoh Laboratories
1670 Oak Ridge Turnpike
Oak Ridge, TN 37830
Phone: 800-292-4794
Fax: 423-481-0799

**LaSalle University School
of Nursing**
1900 W. Olney Ave.
Philadelphia, PA 19038
Phone 215-951-1982
Fax: 215-951-1896

**The Learning Curve
Weingart Designs**
4614 Prospect Ave., #421
Cleveland, OH 44103-4314
Phone: 216-881-5151

LLL Around the World
Contact: Beryl Nielson
46 Marina Vista Ave.
Larkspur, CA 94939

Loving Moms
P.O. Box 147
Skokie, IL 60076-0147
Phone: 800-568-4648

MaMo Designs
133 Kirk Crossing
Decatur, GA 30030
Phone: 404-377-4728

**Maternal and Child Health
Interorganizational Nutrition
Group**
U.S. Department of Health and
Human Services
Public Health Service
Rockville, MD 20857
Phone: 301-594-1360

Maternal Concepts™
P.O. Box 39
Spring Valley, WI 54767
Phone: 715-778-4723/800-310-5817

Medela
P.O. Box 660
McHenry, IL 60051-0660
Phone: 800-435-8316
Fax: 815-363-1246

Medical Center of Delaware
Christiana Hospital
4755 Agletown-Stanton Road
P.O. Box 6001
Newark, DE 19718
Phone: 302-733-2340

Midwifery Today
P.O. Box 2672-316
Eugene, OR 97402
Phone: 800-743-0974
Fax: 541-344-1422
midwifery@AOL.com

**Mothers' Milk Bank
Columbia Presbyterian/St. Luke's
Medical Center**
1719 E. 19th Ave.
Denver, CO 80218
Phone: 303-869-1888
Fax: 303-869-2490

**Mothers' Milk Bank
Valley Medical Center**
751 South Bascom Ave.
San Jose, CA 95128
Phone: 408-998-4550
Fax: 408-885-7381–MMB

**National Alliance for Breastfeeding
Advocacy**
Contact: Barbara Heiser
9684 Oak Hill Dr.
Ellicott City, MD 21043
Phone: 410-995-3726
Fax: 410-992-1977
barbb13@AOL. com

**National Association of WIC
Directors Committee on
Breastfeeding Promotion**
Kathy Dugas, R.D., Chairperson
c/o Mississippi WIC Program
2423 N. State St.
Underwood Annex
Rm. 211
Jackson, MS 39215

**National Capital Lactation Center
and Community Human Milk Bank**
Georgetown University Hospital
3800 Reservoir Rd., N.W.
Washington, DC 20007-2197
Phone: 202-784-6455
Fax: 202-784-2505

National Child Nutrition Project
1501 Cherry St.
Philadelphia, PA 19102

National Maternal and Child Health Clearinghouse
3520 Prospect St., N.W.
Washington, DC 20057

**Nursing Mothers Committee
Family Centered Parents, Inc.**
P.O. Box 142
Rockland, DE 19732

Nursing Mothers Council, Inc.
P.O. Box 50063
Palo Alto, CA 94303
Phone: 408-272-1448

Nursing Mothers Association of Australia (NMAA)
P.O. Box 231
Nunawading, Victoria 3131
Australia
Phone: 61-3-877-5011

Parenting Concepts
P.O. Box 1437
Lake Arrowhead, CA 92352
Phone: 800-727-3683 / 909-337-1499
Fax: 909-337-0969
http://www.comehere.com/P.concept/P.Chome.hpml

Perinatal Center of the University of Leipzig
Sudhang 4
Porta Westfalica 32457
Germany
Phone: 49-571-710618
Fax: 49-571-76921

Pharmasoft Medical Publishing
4606 Oregon
Amarillo, TX 79109
Phone: 800-378-1317 / 806-358-8138

Population Council
One Dag Hammarskjold Plaza
New York, NY 10017

Presbyterian/St. Luke's Medical Center
Lactation Program
1719 E. 19th Ave.
Denver CO 80218
Phone: 303-869-1881
Fax: 303-869-1958

Regional Milk Bank
at Memorial Hospital/Medical Center
of Central Massachusetts
119 Belmont Street
Worcester, MA 01605
Phone: 508-793-6005
Fax: 508-793-6593

Resources for Lactation Professionals
1900 Covington Rd.
Ann Arbor, MI 48103

**Rocky Mountain Poison
and Drug Center**
Drugs in Lactation
8802 E. 9th Ave., Bldg. 752
Denver, CO 80220
Phone: 303-739-1100/900-285-3784
(fee for service)
Fax: 303-739-1119

**Seattle-King County Department
of Public Health**
Breastfeeding Publications
110 Prefontaine Ave. S., Suite 500
Seattle, WA 98104
Phone: 206-296-4774

Shiloh Books
910 Wood St.
Pittsburgh, PA 15221
Phone: 412-371-8844

**Texas Department of Health
and Healthy Mothers, Healthy Babies**
1100 W. 49th St.
Austin, TX 78756
Phone: 512-406-0744
Fax: 512-406-0722
jrourke@wicsc.tdh.state.tx.us
jstremler@wicsc.tdh.state.tx.us

9411 Parkfield, Suite 310
Austin, TX 78758
Phone: 512-719-3010
Fax: 512-719-3011
jfisherrn@aol.com

**Triangle Lactation Center
and Mothers' Milk Bank**
Wake Medical Center
11608 Rutledge Bay
Raleigh, NC 27614
Phone: 919-250-8599
Fax: 919-250-7749
dtully@ral.mindspring.com

**UCLA Extension and UCLA School
of Nursing**
10995 Le Conte Ave., Room 711
Los Angeles, CA 90024
Phone: 310-825-9187
Fax: 310-825-6906
emcnamee@unex.ucla.edu

UNICEF
Nutrition Cluster (H8F)
3 United Nations Plaza
New York, NY 10017
Fax: 212-303-7911

**University of California, San Diego Extension/
Ed Vantage Department**
9500 Gilman Dr., Mail Code 0176
La Jolla, CA 92093-0176
Phone: 619-534-0835
Fax: 619-534-7385

**University of New Mexico
Division of Continuing Education
and Community Services**
Nursing's Allied Health Professional
Development Program
1634 University Blvd., N.E.
Albuquerque, NM 87106
Phone: 505-277-3905
Fax: 505-277-8975
clesper@unm.edu

University of Rochester Medical Center
Department of Pediatrics
Box 777
Rochester, NY 14642
Phone: 716-275-0088
Fax: 716-461-3614

U.S. Committee for UNICEF
Office of Public Policy and Government
Relations
110 Maryland Ave., N.E., Box 36
Washington, DC 20002

**Wake Area Health Education Center
Wake Medical Center
Department of Environment, Health
and Natural Resources**
Lactation Consultants of North Carolina
11608 Rutledge Bay
Raleigh, NC 27614
Phone: 919-847-4903
Fax: 919-250-7749

Wellstart International
4062 First Ave.
San Diego, CA 92103
Phone: 619-295-5192
Fax: 619-294-7787
afulcher@mcimail.com
gwoodwardlopez@mcimail.com

Wichita General Hospital
1600 Eighth St.
Wichita Falls, TX 76301
Phone: 817-761-8536

**Women's International Public
Health Network**
7100 Oak Forest Lane
Bethesda, MD 20817
Phone: 301-469-9211
Fax: 301-469-8423

**World Alliance for Breastfeeding Action
(WABA)**
Contact: Anwar Fazal, WABA Secretariat
P. O. Box 1200
10850 Penang, Malaysia
Phone: 60-4-884-816

World Health Organization (WHO)
WHO Publications Center USA
49 Sheridan Ave.
Albany, NY 12210
Phone: 516-436-9686

References

American Academy of Pediatrics (AAP) (1982). The promotion of breast-feeding. *Pediatrics*, 69:654-61.

AAP (1985). *Pediatric Nutrition Handbook*. AAP: Elk Grove Village, IL.

AAP (1993). AAP policy on direct formula advertising to the public. *AAP News*, 9:2.

AAP/American College of Obstetricians and Gynecologists (ACOG) (1988). *Guidelines for Perinatal Care*, 2nd ed. AAP: Elk Grove Village, IL.

AAP/ACOG (1992). *Guidelines for Perinatal Care*, 3rd ed. AAP: Elk Grove Village, IL.

AAP, Committee on Nutrition (1976). Commentary on breastfeeding and infant formulas. *Pediatrics*, 57:278.

AAP, Committee on Nutrition (1980). Encouraging breastfeeding. *Pediatrics*, 65:657.

AAP, Committee on Nutrition (1992). The use of whole cow's milk in infancy. *Pediatrics*, 89:1105-09.

AAP, Committee on Nutrition and Canadian Paediatric Society (CPS), Nutrition Committee (1978). Breastfeeding: A commentary in celebration of the international year of the child. *Pediatrics*, 62:591-601.

American Dietetic Association (1993). Position of the American Dietetic Association: Promotion and support of breastfeeding. *J Am Diet Assoc*, 93:467-69.

Association of Women's Health, Obstetrics, and Neonatal Nurses (1992). AWHONN position statement. *NAACOG Newsletter*, 19.

Bergevin, Y, Dougherty, C, Kramer, SM (1983). Do infant formula samples shorten the duration of breastfeeding? *Lancet*, 1148-51.

Best, LJ (1991). Components of a comprehensive hospital-based breastfeeding support program. *Breastfeeding Abst*, 7(3):1-2.

Breunig, S, Brady, C (1992). The Florida breastfeeding promotion project: A coalition effort to improve hospital practices and policies. *J Hum Lact*, 8:213-15.

Breunig, S, Merwin, M (1990). *Model Hospital Policies and Protocols to Support Breastfeeding Mothers*. Florida Healthy Mother, Healthy Babies Coalition: Gainesville.

Brown, KH, et al. (1986). Milk consumption and hydration status of exclusively breastfed babies in a warm climate. *J Pediatr*, 108:677-80.

DeCarvalho, M, Klaus, MH, Merkat, RB (1982). Frequency of breastfeeding and serum bilirubin concentration. *Am J Dis Child*, 136:737-38.

Healthy Mothers, Healthy Babies (HMHB) National Coalition (1994). *Baby Friendly Hospital Initiative Feasiblity Study, Executive Summary of the Final Report* (pp. 1-8).

Innocenti Declaration (1990). *On the Protection, Promotion and Support of Breastfeeding*, pp. 1-2. Florence, Italy.

Institute of Medicine (IOM), National Academy of Sciences (NAS) (1990). *Nutrition During Pregnancy*. National Academy Press: Washington, DC.

IOM, NAS (1991). *Nutrition During Lactation*. National Academy Press: Washington, DC.

IOM, NAS (1992a). *Nutrition Services in Perinatal Care*. National Academy Press: Washington, DC.

IOM, NAS (1992b). *Nutrition During Pregnancy and Lactation: An Implementation Guide*. National Academy Press: Washington, DC.

International Baby Food Action Network (IBFAN), International Organization of Consumer Unions (IOCU) (1990). *Protecting Infant Health—A Health Worker's Guide to the International Code of Marketing of Breastmilk Substitutes*, 6th ed. IBFAN/IOCU: Penang, Malaysia.

International Board of Lactation Consultant Examiners (IBLCE) (1996). IBLCE program brochure. IBLCE: Falls Church, VA.

International Childbirth Education Association (ICEA) (1992). ICEA position paper: Infant feeding. *Int J Child Educ*, 7:13-16.

International Lactation Consultant Association (ILCA) (1991). *Position Paper on Infant Feeding*. ILCA: Chicago.

ILCA (1992). *Summary of Hazards of Infant Formula*. ILCA: Chicago.

Jelliffe, DB, Jelliffe, EFP (1988). *Programmes to Promote Breastfeeding*. Oxford University Press: Oxford.

Kearney, MH (1988). Identifying psychosocial obstacles to breastfeeding success. *JOGNN*, 98:105.

Kearney, MH, Cronenwett, LR, Barrett, JA (1990). Breastfeeding problems in the first week postpartum. *Nurs Res*, 39:90-95.

Klaus, MH, Kennell, JH (1976). *Maternal–Infant Bonding*. Mosby: St Louis.

La Leche League International (LLLI) (1991). *The Womanly Art of Breastfeeding*, 35th anniversary ed. LLLI: Schaumburg, IL.

Mohrbacher, N, Stock, J (1996). *The Breastfeeding Answer Book*, 2nd Ed. LLLI: Franklin Park, IL.

National Association of WIC Directors (NAWD) (1989). *Position of National Association of WIC Directors on Breastfeeding Promotion in the WIC Program*. NAWD: Washington, DC.

Ostler, CW (1979). Initial feeding time of newborn infants: Effects upon first meconium passage and serum, indirect bilirubin levels. *Issues Health-care Women*, 1:2-23.

Reiff, MI, Essock-Vitale, SM (1985). Hospital influences on early infant-feeding practices. *Pediatrics*, 76.

Riordan, J, Auerbach, KG (1993). *Breastfeeding and Human Lactation*. Jones and Bartlett: Boston.

Sachdev, HPS, et al. (1991). Water supplementation in exclusively breastfed infants during summer in the tropics. *Lancet*, 337:929-33.

United Nations Children's Fund (UNICEF) (1985). *State of the World's Children*. UNICEF: New York.

U.S. Committee for UNICEF (1994). *Barriers and Solutions to the Global Ten Steps to Successful Breastfeeding: A Summary of In-Depth Interviews with Hospitals Participating in the WHO/UNICEF Baby Friendly Hospital Initiative Interim Program in the United States* (pp. 2-31). U.S. Committee for UNICEF: Washington, DC.

U.S. Department of Health and Human Services (USDHHS) (1984). *Report of the Surgeon General's Workshop on Breastfeeding and Human Lactation*. National Center for Education in Maternal and Child Health: Washington, DC.

USDHHS (1985). *Followup Report: The Surgeon General's Workshop on Breastfeeding and Human Lactation*. National Center for Education in Maternal and Child Health: Washington, DC.

USDHHS (1991). *Second Followup Report: The Surgeon General's Workshop on Breastfeeding and Human Lactation*. National Center for Education in Maternal and Child Health: Washington, DC.

Winikoff, B, Baer, EC (1980). The obstetrician's opportunity: Translating "breast is best" from theory to practice. *Am J Obstet Gynecol*, 138:423-33.

Winikoff, B, Myers, D, Laukaran, VH, Stone, R (1987). Overcoming obstacles to breastfeeding in a large municipal hospital: Applications of lessons learned. *Pediatrics*, 80:423-33.

Woessner, C, Launers, J, Bernard B (1991). *Breastfeeding Today. A Mother's Companion*. Avery Publishing: Garden City, NY, p. 60.

Woolridge, MW, Greasley, V, Silipisornkosol, S (1985). The initiation of lactation: The effect of early versus delayed contact for suckling on milk intake in the first week postpartum: A study in Chiang Mai, Northern Thailand. *Early Hum Dev*, 12(3):269-78.

World Alliance for Breastfeeding Action (WABA) (1992). What you can do to assure your neighborhood hospital or health facility is baby friendly! *The Baby Friendly Hospital Initiative Action Folder*. WABA: Penang, Malaysia.

World Health Organization (WHO) (1981). Resolution of the 34th World Health Assembly, International Code of Marketing of Breastmilk Substitutes, Fifteenth Plenary Meeting.

WHO (1990). *Bulletin of the World Health Organization: Infant Feeding, The Physiological Basis*. WHO: Geneva.

WHO (1994). Resolution of the 47th World Health Assembly, International Code of Marketing of Breastmilk Substitutes, Plenary Meeting.

WHO/UNICEF (1989) *Protecting, Promoting and Supporting Breast-Feeding: The Special Role of Maternity Services*. A Joint WHO/UNICEF Statement. WHO: Geneva.

ADDITIONAL READINGS

Auerbach, KG, Pessyl, MM (1992). A baby-friendly environment: More than a dream? *J Hum Lact*, 8:189-92.

Dungy, CI, Christensen-Szalanski, J, Losch, M, Russell, D (1992). Effect of discharge samples on duration of breastfeeding. *Pediatrics*, 90:233-37.

Eiger, MS (1988). The lactation clinic at Beth Israel Medical Center. *Breastfeeding Abst*, 8(2).

Lamb, ME (1983). Early mother–neonate contact and the mother–child relationship. *J Child Psychol* and *Psych Allied Discip*, 24:487-94.

Lauwers, J, Woessner, C, CEA of Greater Philadelphia (1983). *Counseling the Nursing Mother—A Reference Handbook for Health-Care Providers and Lay Counselors*. Avery Publishing Group: Wayne, NJ.

Lawrence, R (1994). *Breastfeeding: A Guide for the Medical Profession*. Mosby: St. Louis.

Levine, RE, Huffman, SL, Labbok, MH (1990). *Changing Hospital Practices to Promote Breastfeeding: Financial Considerations*. Institute for Reproductive Health, Georgetown University: Washington, DC.

Marmet, C (1993). Summary of institutional actions affecting breastfeeding. *J Hum Lact*, 9:109-12.

Nylander, G, Lindemann, R, Helsing, E, Bendvold, E (1991). Unsupplemented breastfeeding in the maternity ward. *Acta Obstet Gynecol Scand*, 70:205-9.

Righard, L, Alade, MO (1990). Effect of delivery room routines on success of first breastfeed. *Lancet*, 336:1105-7.

Strembel, S, Sass, S, Cole, G, Hartner, J, Fischer, C (1991). Breast-feeding policies and routines among Arizona hospitals and nursery staff: Results and implications of a descriptive study. *J Am Diet Assoc*, 91:923-25.

Suiton, CW, Oslon, JC, Wilson, J (1993). Nutrition care during pregnancy and lactation. *J Am Diet Assoc*, 9:478-79.

Thompson, ME, et al. (1989). The importance of immediate postnatal contact: Its effect on breastfeeding. *Can Fam Physician*, 25:64-66.

Woessner, C (1991). Sending mixed signals: The effects of formula discharge packs. *Breastfeeding Adv*, 2.

Pre- and Post-Test Answer Keys

Breastfeeding in Today's Culture

Pre-Test	Post-Test
1. D	1. B
2. A	2. A
3. D	3. D
4. B	4. B
5. D	5. B
6. B	6. C
7. E	7. A
8. D	8. D
9. A	9. B
10. C	10. C
11. B	11. B
12. D	12. D
13. D	13. C
14. A	14. D
15. C	15. D
16. E	16. A
17. B	17. C
18. C	18. C
19. E	19. E
20. A	20. A

The Impact of Breastfeeding on the Family and Community

Pre-Test	Post-Test
1. A	1. B
2. C	2. B
3. C	3. C
4. D	4. C
5. A	5. A
6. B	6. B
7. B	7. A
8. A	8. B
9. A	9. A
10. B	10. A
11. A	11. B
12. B	12. B
13. D	13. A
14. C	14. B
15. B	15. C
16. A	16. A
17. B	17. A
18. B	18. B
19. A	19. A
20. A	20. B

Prolonging Lactation		Advantages of Breastfeeding	
Pre-Test	**Post-Test**	**Pre-Test**	**Post-Test**
1. B	1. C	1. B	1. B
2. C	2. D	2. D	2. B
3. C	3. C	3. A	3. C
4. B	4. C	4. D	4. B
5. B	5. A	5. C	5. D
6. B	6. B	6. C	6. C
7. A	7. A	7. E	7. A
8. B	8. A	8. B	8. D
9. B	9. B	9. A	9. B
10. A	10. B	10. D	10. E
11. B	11. B	11. C	11. B
12. C	12. A	12. D	12. D
13. A	13. C	13. D	13. B
14. A	14. D	14. E	14. D
15. E	15. E	15. B	15. B
16. B	16. A	16. D	16. A
17. B	17. B	17. A	17. C
18. C	18. A	18. A	18. A
19. A	19. B	19. B	19. B
20. C	20. C	20. E	20. E

Hazards of Artificial Feeding

Pre-Test	Post-Test
1. A	1. D
2. A	2. A
3. D	3. B
4. D	4. D
5. A	5. A
6. C	6. A
7. A	7. B
8. A	8. A
9. E	9. A
10. C	10. E
11. B	11. A
12. A	12. D
13. A	13. A
14. B	14. A
15. A	15. B
16. D	16. C
17. A	17. A
18. B	18. A
19. D	19. A
20. C	20. A

The Promotion of Breastfeeding with Supportive Policies

Pre-Test	Post-Test
1. A	1. C
2. A	2. B
3. B	3. C
4. B	4. C
5. A	5. D
6. B	6. B
7. B	7. B
8. B	8. B
9. A	9. B
10. A	10. A
11. E	11. D
12. D	12. D
13. B	13. B
14. A	14. B
15. D	15. D
16. D	16. A
17. D	17. E
18. A	18. D
19. A	19. D
20. A	20. A

Organizational Positions
Supportive of Breastfeeding

Pre-Test	Post-Test
1. A	1. A
2. A	2. A
3. A	3. A
4. B	4. A
5. A	5. B
6. A	6. A
7. B	7. A
8. A	8. A
9. A	9. A
10. B	10. B
11. B	11. A
12. A	12. A
13. A	13. A
14. A	14. A
15. A	15. B
16. B	16. A
17. A	17. B
18. A	18. B
19. A	19. A
20. A	20. A

How to Receive Continuing Education Credits

The four individual modules of the *Lactation Specialist Self-Study Series* have been approved for continuing education hours/continuing education recognition points (CERPs)/contact hours from the following organizations:

Commission on Dietetic Registration (CDR): The credentialing agency for the American Dietetic Association.

Georgia Nurses Association (GNA): The Georgia Nurses Association is accredited as an Approver of Continuing Education in Nursing by the American Nurses Credentialing Center Commission on Accreditation.

International Board of Lactation Consultant Examiners (IBLCE): The International Board of Lactation Consultant Examiners is the credentialing agency for the International Lactation Consultant Association.

The individual purchasing the module(s) can apply for continuing education credits/contact hours/CERPs for any **one** or **all** of the four modules in the series. The following chart explains the credits approved by each organization for each of the four modules:

		CDR*	GNA	IBLCE
Module 1	*The Support of Breastfeeding*	15 CE Category II	18	18L Independent
Module 2	*The Process of Breastfeeding*	15 CE Category III	18	18L Independent
Module 3	*The Science of Breastfeeding*	23 CE Category III	27	27L Independent
Module 4	*The Management of Breastfeeding*	15 CE Category III	18	18L Independent

*The commission on Dietetic Registration has approved all four modules for specialist CE approval for Board Certified Specialists in Pediatric Nutrition.

Procedure to Follow to Apply for Credits

Step 1   Remove the application for continuing education, answer sheet and evaluation from the back of the module. Do not lose the application form as it has been specially processed to identify originals packaged with each module and can only be replaced for a $25.00 fee accompanied by the original receipt of purchase. Photocopies of the application form will not be accepted. Only one application is needed to apply for credits from more than one organization. Complete the application for continuing education.

Step 2   Review the objectives for each section prior to reading the section or taking the pre-test. Take the pre-test and fill in your answers on the answer sheet for the section to be studied. You must complete the pre-test to obtain credits although your score on the pre-test will not influence whether or not you obtain credits. Please answer the pre-test to the best of your ability as the score on the pre-test will be pooled with the scores from other applicants to assist the editors in identifying areas applicants are weak in and will be compared to your post-test to quantify the success of the module in enhancing learning.

After you have taken the pre-test and recorded your answers on the official answer sheet, read and study the section. Finally, complete the post-test and fill in the answers on the official answer sheet. **Only the answers on the post-test will be scored**. You must receive a 70% correct on the post-test for each section in the module to obtain credit. If you score less than 70% on any one post-test of the module you will be sent a listing of references pertinent to the section(s) you did not complete successfully and can re-apply for continuing education credits for a discounted fee of $1.00 per continuing education credit. Should this occur, you will be sent another answer sheet to use as photocopies of the answer sheets are not accepted.

Step 3   Complete the module evaluation after reading each section. The module evaluations will be analyzed and the information obtained used to improve and enhance the series. Send the module evaluation(s), official answer sheets(s) and check, money order or credit card information to ANC, Inc. 4571-A Cox Road, Evans, Georgia 30809.

Allow three weeks for processing. Rush processing is available for an extra $25.00 and scoring and notification of credits to credentialing agencies will be completed within three business days of receiving your application.

Step 4   Upon successful completion of all of the post-tests for a module, you will be sent a certificate of completion for each organization that you have requested credit from, your name will be forwarded to the appropriate credentialing organization if appropriate, and a record will be maintained of your successful completion for five years. Requests for duplicate certificates can be honored for a processing fee of $10.00.

Module 1   The Support of Breastfeeding
APPLICATION FOR CONTINUING EDUCATION

Name _____ Address _____
As it will appear on certificate   Street, Rural Route, or Post Office Box

City _____ State or Province _____ Zip Code _____

Country _____

Daytime Phone Number _____ E-Mail _____
Area Code and Number

Please complete the information for the organization(s) from whom you are requesting credits:

Commission on Dietetic Registration   CE hours: __ × \$2.00 = _____

Board Certified Specialist in Pediatric Nutrition   Yes or No

Registration Number _____

Georgia Nurses Association   Contact hours: __ × \$2.00 = _____

SSN/SIN _____

International Board of Lactation   CERPs: __ × \$2.00 = _____
Consultant Examiners

SSN/SIN or IBLCE nine-digit ID number _____

Optional rush processing (\$25.00 fee) _____

TOTAL _____

Checks, money orders and credit cards accepted.

No purchase orders.

____ MasterCard ____ Visa ____ American Express

Account Number _____ Expiration Date _____

Name as it appears on the card _____

Checks or money orders may be made out to **Augusta Nutrition Consultants, Inc. (ANC)** and sent with the evaluation and the completed answer sheet to 4571-A Cox Road, Evans, Georgia 30809. DO NOT SEND TO JONES AND BARTLETT PUBLISHERS.

Note: You must submit this **original** form to receive continuing education units. Photocopies cannot be accepted.

Evaluation
The Support of Breastfeeding

Please comment on the degree of content difficulty, effectiveness of learning method, and objectives for the following topics by putting a checkmark next to the response that best describes the material.

Breastfeeding in Today's Culture

Content level	○ too high	○ appropriate	○ too low
Effectiveness of learning method	○ excellent/very good	○ good	○ fair/poor
Information	○ useful		○ not useful

Use the following key for the objectives and circle your response:

1 = STRONGLY MET   **2** = MET   **3** = SOMEWHAT MET   **4** = SOMEWHAT NOT MET   **5** = NOT MET

At the completion of this section, the learner will be able to do the following:

1. Describe the factors that contributed to the rise of the artificial baby milk industry.   1 2 3 4 5

2. Discuss the impact of socially determined attitudes on women's choice to breastfeed.   1 2 3 4 5

3. Describe the demographics of who breastfeeds in the United States.   1 2 3 4 5

4. Differentiate among patterns and trends in infant feeding in the U.S. population as a whole, the WIC population, and the world population.   1 2 3 4 5

5. Discuss the factors important in the decision to breastfeed.   1 2 3 4 5

6. Describe the barriers to breastfeeding in different population groups.   1 2 3 4 5

7. Describe counseling strategies that mey be effective in removing barriers.   1 2 3 4 5

8. Identify common myths about breastfeeding prevalent in the United States.   1 2 3 4 5

9. Write a marketing plan to promote a product or service related to breastfeeding.   1 2 3 4 5

The Impact of Breastfeeding on the Family and Community

Content level   ○ too high   ○ appropriate   ○ too low

Effectiveness of learning method   ○ excellent/very good   ○ good   ○ fair/poor

Information   ○ useful   ○ not useful

Use the following key for the objectives and circle your response:

1 = STRONGLY MET   **2** = MET   **3** = SOMEWHAT MET   **4** = SOMEWHAT NOT MET   **5** = NOT MET

At the completion of this section, the learner will be able to do the following:

1. Discuss the changes in family relationships that occur with the birth of a child.   1 2 3 4 5

2. Discuss the impact of breastfeeding on the father and describe his role in caring for the mother-infant dyad.   1 2 3 4 5

3. Discuss extended family members' roles and concerns when breastfeeding is the infant feeding choice.   1 2 3 4 5

4. Discuss the difficulties that returning to work after the birth of a baby can present for the breastfeeding family.   1 2 3 4 5

5. Describe practical suggestions to ease the transition to work for the breastfeeding family.   1 2 3 4 5

Prolonging Lactation

Content level   ○ too high   ○ appropriate   ○ too low

Effectiveness of learning method   ○ excellent/very good   ○ good   ○ fair/poor

Information   ○ useful   ○ not useful

Use the following key for the objectives and circle your response:

1 = STRONGLY MET   **2** = MET   **3** = SOMEWHAT MET   **4** = SOMEWHAT NOT MET   **5** = NOT MET

At the completion of this section, the learner will be able to do the following:

1. Discuss why prolonging the duration of breastfeeding is important.   1 2 3 4 5

2. Discuss the factors influencing breastfeeding duration.   1 2 3 4 5

3. Describe community and governmental support programs available for breastfeeding families.   1 2 3 4 5

4. Discuss the role of the lactation consultant and other health-care profesionals in supporting breastfeeding.   1 2 3 4 5

5. Discuss the legal rights of breastfeeding families.   1 2 3 4 5

Advantages of Breastfeeding

Content level	○ too high	○ appropriate	○ too low
Effectiveness of learning method	○ excellent/very good	○ good	○ fair/poor
Information	○ useful		○ not useful

Use the following key for the objectives and circle your response:

1 = STRONGLY MET   **2** = MET   **3** = SOMEWHAT MET   **4** = SOMEWHAT NOT MET   **5** = NOT MET

At the completion of this section, the learner will be able to do the following:

1. Discuss four infant benefits from breastfeeding.   1 2 3 4 5

2. Discuss two maternal benefits from breastfeeding.   1 2 3 4 5

3. Discuss three benefits to society from breastfeeding.   1 2 3 4 5

Hazards of Artificial Feeding

Content level	○ too high	○ appropriate	○ too low
Effectiveness of learning method	○ excellent/very good	○ good	○ fair/poor
Information	○ useful		○ not useful

Use the following key for the objectives and circle your response:

1 = STRONGLY MET   **2** = MET   **3** = SOMEWHAT MET   **4** = SOMEWHAT NOT MET   **5** = NOT MET

At the completion of this section, the learner will be able to do the following:

1. Discuss four hazards of artificial feeding to the infant.   1 2 3 4 5

2. Name two infections the infant is at increased risk for contract-   1 2 3 4 5
   ing if artificially fed.

3. Discuss information that must be provided to parents so an   1 2 3 4 5
   informed decision can be made.

The Promotion of Breastfeeding with Supportive Policies

Content level   ○ too high   ○ appropriate   ○ too low

Effectiveness of   ○ excellent/very good   ○ good   ○ fair/poor
learning method

Information   ○ useful   ○ not useful

Use the following key for the objectives and circle your response:

1 = STRONGLY MET   **2** = MET   **3** = SOMEWHAT MET   **4** = SOMEWHAT NOT MET   **5** = NOT MET

At the completion of this section, the learner will be able to do the following:

1. State the effects of the health-care professional's attitude,   1 2 3 4 5
   routines, verbal and nonverbal responses toward influencing
   the decision of a mother to breastfeed and her success.

2. Discuss the national breastfeeding objective adopted by the   1 2 3 4 5
   U.S. Surgeon General at the 1984 Surgeon General's Work-
   shop on Breastfeeding and Human Lactation.

3. Describe practices that discourage breastfeeding.   1 2 3 4 5

4. Identify strategies that will encourage and support the initia-   1 2 3 4 5
   tion of breastfeeding.

5. Explain how implementing the WHO/UNICEF Ten Steps to   1 2 3 4 5
   Successful Breastfeeding statement lays a foundation for the
   implementation and continuation of a successful breastfeeding experience.

Organizational Positions Supportive of Breastfeeding

Content level   ○ too high   ○ appropriate   ○ too low

Effectiveness of   ○ excellent/very good   ○ good   ○ fair/poor
learning method

Information   ○ useful   ○ not useful

Use the following key for the objectives and circle your response:

1 = STRONGLY MET   **2** = MET   **3** = SOMEWHAT MET   **4** = SOMEWHAT NOT MET   **5** = NOT MET

At the completion of this section, the learner will be able to do the following:

1. Descuss professional positions regarding the promotion of   1 2 3 4 5
   breastfeeding as provided in policy statements.

Describe how the information presented is applicable to your practice:

Please tell us what you liked the best about the material:

Please tell us what you liked the least about the material:

Please evaluate the time required to complete the module when compared to the continuing education hours offered:

more time required than hours awarded

approximately the same time required as hours awarded

less time required than hours awarded

Additional Comments:

Module 1 *The Support of Breastfeeding* Answer Sheet

Please use a number-2 pencil to darken your response.

Chapter 1 Section A
Breastfeeding in Today's Culture

	Pre-Test						Post-Test				
	a	b	c	d	e		a	b	c	d	e
1.	O	O	O	O	O	1.	O	O	O	O	O
2.	O	O	O	O	O	2.	O	O	O	O	O
3.	O	O	O	O	O	3.	O	O	O	O	O
4.	O	O	O	O	O	4.	O	O	O	O	O
5.	O	O	O	O	O	5.	O	O	O	O	O
6.	O	O	O	O	O	6.	O	O	O	O	O
7.	O	O	O	O	O	7.	O	O	O	O	O
8.	O	O	O	O	O	8.	O	O	O	O	O
9.	O	O	O	O	O	9.	O	O	O	O	O
10.	O	O	O	O	O	10.	O	O	O	O	O
11.	O	O	O	O	O	11.	O	O	O	O	O
12.	O	O	O	O	O	12.	O	O	O	O	O
13.	O	O	O	O	O	13.	O	O	O	O	O
14.	O	O	O	O	O	14.	O	O	O	O	O
15.	O	O	O	O	O	15.	O	O	O	O	O
16.	O	O	O	O	O	16.	O	O	O	O	O
17.	O	O	O	O	O	17.	O	O	O	O	O
18.	O	O	O	O	O	18.	O	O	O	O	O
19.	O	O	O	O	O	19.	O	O	O	O	O
20.	O	O	O	O	O	20.	O	O	O	O	O

Chapter 1 Section B   The Impact of
Breastfeeding on the Family and Community

	Pre-Test						Post-Test				
	a	b	c	d	e		a	b	c	d	e
1.	O	O	O	O	O	1.	O	O	O	O	O
2.	O	O	O	O	O	2.	O	O	O	O	O
3.	O	O	O	O	O	3.	O	O	O	O	O
4.	O	O	O	O	O	4.	O	O	O	O	O
5.	O	O	O	O	O	5.	O	O	O	O	O
6.	O	O	O	O	O	6.	O	O	O	O	O
7.	O	O	O	O	O	7.	O	O	O	O	O
8.	O	O	O	O	O	8.	O	O	O	O	O
9.	O	O	O	O	O	9.	O	O	O	O	O
10.	O	O	O	O	O	10.	O	O	O	O	O
11.	O	O	O	O	O	11.	O	O	O	O	O
12.	O	O	O	O	O	12.	O	O	O	O	O
13.	O	O	O	O	O	13.	O	O	O	O	O
14.	O	O	O	O	O	14.	O	O	O	O	O
15.	O	O	O	O	O	15.	O	O	O	O	O
16.	O	O	O	O	O	16.	O	O	O	O	O
17.	O	O	O	O	O	17.	O	O	O	O	O
18.	O	O	O	O	O	18.	O	O	O	O	O
19.	O	O	O	O	O	19.	O	O	O	O	O
20.	O	O	O	O	O	20.	O	O	O	O	O

Chapter 1 Section C
Prolonging Lactation

Chapter 2 Section A
Advantages of Breastfeeding

	Pre-Test						**Post-Test**				
	a	b	c	d	e		a	b	c	d	e
1.	O	O	O	O	O	1.	O	O	O	O	O
2.	O	O	O	O	O	2.	O	O	O	O	O
3.	O	O	O	O	O	3.	O	O	O	O	O
4.	O	O	O	O	O	4.	O	O	O	O	O
5.	O	O	O	O	O	5.	O	O	O	O	O
6.	O	O	O	O	O	6.	O	O	O	O	O
7.	O	O	O	O	O	7.	O	O	O	O	O
8.	O	O	O	O	O	8.	O	O	O	O	O
9.	O	O	O	O	O	9.	O	O	O	O	O
10.	O	O	O	O	O	10.	O	O	O	O	O
11.	O	O	O	O	O	11.	O	O	O	O	O
12.	O	O	O	O	O	12.	O	O	O	O	O
13.	O	O	O	O	O	13.	O	O	O	O	O
14.	O	O	O	O	O	14.	O	O	O	O	O
15.	O	O	O	O	O	15.	O	O	O	O	O
16.	O	O	O	O	O	16.	O	O	O	O	O
17.	O	O	O	O	O	17.	O	O	O	O	O
18.	O	O	O	O	O	18.	O	O	O	O	O
19.	O	O	O	O	O	19.	O	O	O	O	O
20.	O	O	O	O	O	20.	O	O	O	O	O

	Pre-Test						**Post-Test**				
	a	b	c	d	e		a	b	c	d	e
1.	O	O	O	O	O	1.	O	O	O	O	O
2.	O	O	O	O	O	2.	O	O	O	O	O
3.	O	O	O	O	O	3.	O	O	O	O	O
4.	O	O	O	O	O	4.	O	O	O	O	O
5.	O	O	O	O	O	5.	O	O	O	O	O
6.	O	O	O	O	O	6.	O	O	O	O	O
7.	O	O	O	O	O	7.	O	O	O	O	O
8.	O	O	O	O	O	8.	O	O	O	O	O
9.	O	O	O	O	O	9.	O	O	O	O	O
10.	O	O	O	O	O	10.	O	O	O	O	O
11.	O	O	O	O	O	11.	O	O	O	O	O
12.	O	O	O	O	O	12.	O	O	O	O	O
13.	O	O	O	O	O	13.	O	O	O	O	O
14.	O	O	O	O	O	14.	O	O	O	O	O
15.	O	O	O	O	O	15.	O	O	O	O	O
16.	O	O	O	O	O	16.	O	O	O	O	O
17.	O	O	O	O	O	17.	O	O	O	O	O
18.	O	O	O	O	O	18.	O	O	O	O	O
19.	O	O	O	O	O	19.	O	O	O	O	O
20.	O	O	O	O	O	20.	O	O	O	O	O

Chapter 2 Section B
Hazards of Artificial Feeding

	Pre-Test						Post-Test				
	a	b	c	d	e		a	b	c	d	e
1.	O	O	O	O	O	1.	O	O	O	O	O
2.	O	O	O	O	O	2.	O	O	O	O	O
3.	O	O	O	O	O	3.	O	O	O	O	O
4.	O	O	O	O	O	4.	O	O	O	O	O
5.	O	O	O	O	O	5.	O	O	O	O	O
6.	O	O	O	O	O	6.	O	O	O	O	O
7.	O	O	O	O	O	7.	O	O	O	O	O
8.	O	O	O	O	O	8.	O	O	O	O	O
9.	O	O	O	O	O	9.	O	O	O	O	O
10.	O	O	O	O	O	10.	O	O	O	O	O
11.	O	O	O	O	O	11.	O	O	O	O	O
12.	O	O	O	O	O	12.	O	O	O	O	O
13.	O	O	O	O	O	13.	O	O	O	O	O
14.	O	O	O	O	O	14.	O	O	O	O	O
15.	O	O	O	O	O	15.	O	O	O	O	O
16.	O	O	O	O	O	16.	O	O	O	O	O
17.	O	O	O	O	O	17.	O	O	O	O	O
18.	O	O	O	O	O	18.	O	O	O	O	O
19.	O	O	O	O	O	19.	O	O	O	O	O
20.	O	O	O	O	O	20.	O	O	O	O	O

Chapter 3 Section A   The Promotion
of Breastfeeding with Supportive Policies

	Pre-Test						Post-Test				
	a	b	c	d	e		a	b	c	d	e
1.	O	O	O	O	O	1.	O	O	O	O	O
2.	O	O	O	O	O	2.	O	O	O	O	O
3.	O	O	O	O	O	3.	O	O	O	O	O
4.	O	O	O	O	O	4.	O	O	O	O	O
5.	O	O	O	O	O	5.	O	O	O	O	O
6.	O	O	O	O	O	6.	O	O	O	O	O
7.	O	O	O	O	O	7.	O	O	O	O	O
8.	O	O	O	O	O	8.	O	O	O	O	O
9.	O	O	O	O	O	9.	O	O	O	O	O
10.	O	O	O	O	O	10.	O	O	O	O	O
11.	O	O	O	O	O	11.	O	O	O	O	O
12.	O	O	O	O	O	12.	O	O	O	O	O
13.	O	O	O	O	O	13.	O	O	O	O	O
14.	O	O	O	O	O	14.	O	O	O	O	O
15.	O	O	O	O	O	15.	O	O	O	O	O
16.	O	O	O	O	O	16.	O	O	O	O	O
17.	O	O	O	O	O	17.	O	O	O	O	O
18.	O	O	O	O	O	18.	O	O	O	O	O
19.	O	O	O	O	O	19.	O	O	O	O	O
20.	O	O	O	O	O	20.	O	O	O	O	O

Chapter 3 Section B　Organizational Positions
Supportive of Breastfeeding

	Pre-Test						**Post-Test**				
	a	b	c	d	e		a	b	c	d	e
1.	O	O	O	O	O	1.	O	O	O	O	O
2.	O	O	O	O	O	2.	O	O	O	O	O
3.	O	O	O	O	O	3.	O	O	O	O	O
4.	O	O	O	O	O	4.	O	O	O	O	O
5.	O	O	O	O	O	5.	O	O	O	O	O
6.	O	O	O	O	O	6.	O	O	O	O	O
7.	O	O	O	O	O	7.	O	O	O	O	O
8.	O	O	O	O	O	8.	O	O	O	O	O
9.	O	O	O	O	O	9.	O	O	O	O	O
10.	O	O	O	O	O	10.	O	O	O	O	O
11.	O	O	O	O	O	11.	O	O	O	O	O
12.	O	O	O	O	O	12.	O	O	O	O	O
13.	O	O	O	O	O	13.	O	O	O	O	O
14.	O	O	O	O	O	14.	O	O	O	O	O
15.	O	O	O	O	O	15.	O	O	O	O	O
16.	O	O	O	O	O	16.	O	O	O	O	O
17.	O	O	O	O	O	17.	O	O	O	O	O
18.	O	O	O	O	O	18.	O	O	O	O	O
19.	O	O	O	O	O	19.	O	O	O	O	O
20.	O	O	O	O	O	20.	O	O	O	O	O